THE PSYCHOLOGY OF
THOUGHT AND FEELING

Founded by

The International Library of Psychology

GENERAL PSYCHOLOGY
In 38 Volumes

THE PSYCHOLOGY OF THOUGHT AND FEELING

A Conservative Interpretation of Results in Modern Psychology

CHARLES PLATT

First published in 1921 by
Routledge, Trench, Trubner & Co., Ltd.

Reprinted in 1999 by
Routledge

2 Park Square, Milton Park, Abingdon, Oxfordshire OX14 4RN
711 Third Avenue, New York, NY 10017
First issued in paperback 2014

Routledge is an imprint of the Taylor and Francis Group, an informa business

Transferred to Digital Printing 2007

© 1921 Charles Platt

British Library Cataloguing in Publication Data
A CIP catalogue record for this book
is available from the British Library

The Psychology of Thought and Feeling

ISBN 978-0-415-21037-9 (hbk)
ISBN 978-0-415-75802-4 (pbk)

General Psychology: 38 Volumes
ISBN 978-0-415-21129-1
The International Library of Psychology: 204 Volumes
ISBN 978-0-415-19132-6

THE PSYCHOLOGY OF
THOUGHT AND FEELING

PREFACE

This book is the outgrowth from a series of lectures, the reception of which has flattered the author into believing that he may, by their publication, satisfy the wants of a larger circle. Such a judgment is, of course, open to suspicion, but the basis for it lies in the fact that psychology, with its wide appeal, has heretofore been treated in its entirety only in the textbook manner. Psychology, while complex, is not abstruse; its conclusions are open to all; no other attributes of mind are required for its understanding than receptivity and common sense. Moreover, its conclusions are too important socially to be neglected in these troublous times, and should be in the possession of all. It is proposed, then, here to give a reasonably complete survey of the whole field, treating the matter briefly, indeed, but, it is hoped, so suggestively that the thought may be led beyond the compass of this small book. The social and educational bearings of the subject will be kept in the foreground throughout, while technicalities and, so far as is possible, controversial and metaphysical problems will be omitted. No Don Quixote ever fought more windmills than has the older school of psychologists. It is the recognition of the windmills, and the agreement to pass them by as unworthy of combat, that is the excuse for this present writing.

Having been prepared originally for lecture purposes, it has been found difficult now to give that careful attention to "authorities" which the written word demands, but effort will be made in the following pages to place credit where due. I take occasion here to express my especial obligation to Dr. Henry Herbert Goddard and to Prof. William McDougall.

Hillbrook,   C. P.
Ardmore, Pa.

CONTENTS

ix

CONTENTS

THE PSYCHOLOGY OF THOUGHT AND FEELING

CHAPTER I

FUNDAMENTAL CONCEPTIONS: ANATOMICAL AND OTHERWISE

MAN, unlike other animals, is curious as to himself. The WHY of his actions, the HOW of his thought, the WHAT of his ego—these are the problems which have ever dangled tantalizingly before him. KNOW THYSELF, commanded the portals of Apollo's temples, and man has ever striven earnestly to obey the behest. Nor has the endeavour been always futile—practical results have been attained even in the philosophical-metaphysical past; Socrates was subtile in analysis; Montaigne, twenty centuries later, was admirable in description; and Browning has been unsurpassed in the expression of intuitive feeling. But, there was something wrong —the problems were too ambitious. With the Ego was sought Consciousness, and, soon, Time, and Space, and the Soul. Abstracts, in general, enveloped the seeker in so dense a mental fog, and led him plunging along so miry a way, that he was able to extricate himself only after abandoning all that he had gained. The metaphysical discussion commonly came out the same road it had entered, or, if it did not so emerge, it remained a mere mental gymnastic of most limited appeal. It would seem that the seeker in metaphysical psychology set out, he the most complex and artificial of men, to study himself by a process of introspection. His effort was to get outside of himself, to study himself from without, but the fact remained that what he studied was that which he studied with. It was a lifting of one's self by the boot-straps, and, as the gentle Philosopher of Chelsea said of it, "a hopeless struggle for the wisest as for the foolishest," adding, by way of pertinent commentary, "an Irish saint once swam the Channel carrying his head in his teeth, but the feat has never been imitated."

Then came Darwin and a new biology. Doors were opened, and psychology timidly peeped through with interested longing glances at the new world revealed. These doors were labelled Ethics, and Morals, Social and Political Economy, Law, Criminology, Medicine, Business, History, and Education—they offered much

2

promise. But no, the psychologist must not venture to pass—the authority of society excitedly prevented. "Our social structures are complete; these doors lead to error." The church shrieked its horror at what had been glimpsed, and law, medicine, and economics, and even pedagogy, quick shut their eyes. With prompt understanding, the Existing-Concepts recognized that what the seeking psychologist was making toward would shake their very foundations. The new thought, then, must of course be wrong; and the psychologist, if he wished to retain his place in society (if he wished, for instance, to retain his chair in the university), must keep hands off. In the face of this universal bow-wow what was the poor student to do? The result, the first product of the possibilities of a broader science, was a retirement from the affairs of society altogether; a withdrawal to the laboratory, and devotion there, of time and thought, to artificial experiment. Psychology became a thing of apparatus and remained barren before the world. Charted curves of reactions took the place of metaphysical discussion, and the result was even less interesting than before. So was psychology one generation ago.

What has brought about the present change?

I do not know, but I suspect the world unrest, and the doubt, beginning to form in man's mind, that all was not so well as had been proclaimed.

The phase which we are now passing through socially may be characterized as the Phase of the Militant Minorities. Now minorities are not always wrong, and whether, with Henry Adams and others, we should apply to society the second law of thermodynamics, the law of the degradation of energy, may still well be doubted, but, on the other hand, such evidence as society can produce would not seem to be very encouraging. Indolent majorities have everywhere bowed to the pathological energies of small abnormal groups. The political economists have seen their well-planned structures tumbled about them, and are even now being driven to explain. It is a time for taking inventory—it is more than this, it is a time when our understanding of affairs must become more real; when man must make a complete readjustment of the social mechanism—"If we do not mend the machine, there are forces moving in the world that will break it." * Possibly— difficult thought!—the existing economies may not have been founded on elemental truth after all!

* Stephen Leacock, *The Unsolved Riddle of Social Justice.*

4

The above is one way of looking at it. There is another. Possibly the machine is all right, and the trouble is with us. Possibly we are not using the machine to advantage, and it is ourselves that need the mending. What we may need is not a readjustment of the social mechanism, but a readjustment to it. At any rate, let us study man once again and not rest on our present formulas. Biology in its investigations seeks the simpler manifestations of a life form, and builds from these to the more complex. Let us do the same. Let us study the child; and let us study man, too, but in the more primitive environment of savagery; and let us study the idiot and the imbecile, whom we may take as the permanent children of the race, willing to stand still while we study. The savage is not necessarily primitive, nor is the imbecile the same as the child, but the relation in each case is a real one, and based upon it is much of the reasoning that follows.

Whatever the cause of the new attitude toward the science, the doors are now flung wide, and psychology has come to its being. What William James defined as "the description and explanation of states of consciousness, as such," William McDougall, in the modern spirit, defines as "the science of behaviour and

of conduct.'' The evolution of the last generation in psychology is seen in these two defini-
tions. The principles of organic evolution, the
facts of anatomy, and the interpretations of
physiology and pathology, are all called into
service, and useful work in practical fields
begins.

.   .   .   .

Let us adopt as a general thesis:—that man
has certain tendencies or dispositions; that
these determine his actions; that most of these
dispositions are innate, inherited, and are, in
one sense, unchangeable; that they may, however, be modified in their expression by education and experience. Further, we will conceive
society, as we find it, to be a product of these
innate tendencies of the individual—a composite of the individuals composing it. And,
finally, we will recognize that while society is
so composed, it, in turn, reacts upon the individual, directing and modifying his every
action. The individual is what he is because
of his innate tendencies as modified by society.
Society—institutions, customs, parties, ideals,
morals, all these—is what it is, under normal
conditions, in response to the needs of the
individual.

It is true that individuals are many, and

types are many, but similar-minded men tend to come together, so that, in fact, society presents not one composite, but many—the composite groups of like-minded. Thus a certain small group of thoughtful people unite to form a Unitarian Fellowship, while a vastly larger group unite to form the Roman Catholic Church. One baby is born a Conservative, another is born a Liberal. And this means far more than just being born into a conservative family, or into a liberal family, or into a Unitarian family; it means, literally, being born with the innate tendencies appropriate to one or the other of these attitudes. It means, too, therefore, though fortunately this does not often happen, that a Unitarian may be born into a Catholic family, or a Catholic into a Unitarian family, or a conservative into a liberal family. I say that it is fortunate that this does not often happen, for when it does it must result either in but lukewarm adherence to the family traditions, or in severance from the same, amid family laments. The accident of birth may determine, at least temporarily, a man's classification, but it is the luggage the baby brings into the world, his potential brain patterns, which will decide what he is really to be.

I have adopted the term innate tendency, or

disposition, where the term *instinct* is commonly used, but this latter word I prefer to reserve for a more specific and limited application. By innate tendency I mean an inherited psychological and physiological disposition which determines that its possessor shall react in a particular manner to a given stimulus. These dispositions will vary all the way from simple nerve reflexes, such as the knee-jerk, to the most highly complex emotional reactions, and in this range, of course, the instincts will be included; but I follow Bergson in making instinct a specific evolutionary product—a diverging tendency, not a linear antecedent of man's intellectuality. This will be referred to later, under sex. It is with the innate tendency in general that we are now concerned, especially with its higher manifestations. It is assumed that the stimulus, being received, excites a prepared brain pattern which, in turn, gives origin to an emotional state. This emotional state may itself rise but faintly into consciousness; but the two together, the brain pattern reinforced by the emotion, result in characteristic action.

The word *pattern* will be frequently used in this book. Let us get, to start with, a clear conception of this convenient term, and for this purpose let me review, in the briefest possible manner, the structure of the nervous system. We shall omit as irrelevant to our aim all the refinements of modern physiological research.

There are in the human body, and in the bodies of all the higher animals, two related systems of nerves, the cerebro-spinal and the sympathetic, the former being directly associated with our voluntary movements, and the latter more intimately associated with the life process itself, and, therefore, with the more involuntary acts of the body.

Starting with the cerebro-spinal system, and its centre, the brain, we find this latter to be a bulk of nerve tissue containing, as its essential elements, myriads of nerve cells from which pass off tentacle-like processes of varying length. There are in all some ten thousand million of these cells, or neurons, as they are called, arranged in certain fairly defined but merging groups, each with its specific function. The brain is placed in a bony compartment, the skull, and is thereby protected from direct interference from without, but it is connected with the rest of the body, and, in a sense, with the external world, by the nerves, the prolongations of the nerve cell processes just mentioned. Certain of these cell processes, the cranial nerves, pass through openings in the skull to the face and neighbouring regions, while others, the spinal nerves, unite to form the cable of the spinal cord, to be later given off to the body at regular intervals through apertures in the spinal column.

The spinal cord itself contains nerve cells, these acting as relays to the transmission of the nerve impulse, much as in telegraphy the electric impulse is carried long distances by means of relay batteries. Thus, a nerve impulse does not pass over a continuous "wire" from the point of stimulation to the receptive area in the brain, but, after travelling a longer or shorter distance, the "wire" is broken, and the impulse picked up and relayed on by another nerve cell. Several such interruptions may occur in the total path.

In this manner the brain is connected with the rest of the body; certain of the nerves carrying *afferent* or incoming currents, and certain others, the *efferent* or outgoing. The afferent nerves carry to the brain stimulations received by their distal extremities; the brain receives this stimulation, reacts in a certain manner, and then sends out an appropriate answer, an impulse over the efferent nerves. Thus, the hand has been placed upon a hot plate

—a stimulus passes over certain nerves, whose function it is to receive impressions of temperature, and this stimulation, reaching the brain, there causes a reaction which results in the activating of certain cells in the motor area. From these motor cells there passes out an impulse over the efferent nerves by which the proper muscles are set in motion, and the hand is withdrawn. In the same manner the stimuli of sight, hearing, smell, touch, pain, and pressure, are brought to the brain, and, there being appreciated, give rise to appropriate action.

In certain nerve actions, notably in those known as *reflex,* it may be that the nerve impulse will not reach the brain until after the action, its purpose, has been already accomplished. Here it would seem that under certain conditions, as, for instance, for safety's sake, where delay would be dangerous, the duty of the brain may be taken over by the nerve cells of the spinal cord, as being usefully nearer to the source of stimulation. Your hand comes into contact with the point of a pin, and it is instantly jerked away, but the pain may not be *felt* until after the action is completed, or at least until after it has been begun. Here the motor impulse was supplied by motor cells in the spinal cord, though the stimulus did still pass on to the brain where it was duly received and registered—in explanation, as it were, of the usurped function. It would seem reasonable to assume that all reflexes have, or have had, a purpose, but some of the reflexes now possessed by man are not explainable by any present known need. They probably remain with us as vestiges of the past. In a general way there has been a tendency in animal development to put more and more of the burden of life on the brain. Many of the functions there seated with us, in less developed animals are performed habitually under the control of the spinal nerve centres. Thus, a frog from which the brain has been removed will still behave much as a perfectly good frog should do. It will "strike out" when placed in water; it will creep up an inclined plane; it will endeavour to brush off a drop of acid placed upon its skin.

James has said that the animal takes in and gives out, while man takes in, turns over, and gives out—the turning-over process being the mental appreciation of a stimulus as an antecedent to action. But, aside from the spinal reflexes common to both man and beast, *both* man and beast do "turn over" in the brain all received stimulation, whether the process be a conscious one or not. All brain action is not necessarily conscious, and many actions styled reflex are really unconscious brain actions—unconscious because so established by habit that they no longer need our attention for their performance. Of these *automatic* actions, as they should properly be called, other animals undoubtedly possess more than does man.

It is to be remembered that in all of this flow of the nerve current, incoming and outgoing, and within the brain itself, the path of the flow becomes frequently broken. The nerve force, the neurokyme, flows through a process of the nerve cell, through the body of the cell, and through another process or extension for a greater or lesser distance, and then comes a break—leaping now a microscopic gap it passes on to the process of another cell to be, in turn, relayed by this on its farther course. *At each of these breaks a choice presents itself*—which of the close-lying neighbouring cells shall it be that shall pick up the current and thus pass it on? It is here that the innate disposition steps in. The evolutionary development itself has determined in a general way the direction of the nerve path, but its minor deviations depend upon the particular inheritances of the individual.

Now a path once travelled is the path most easily retravelled. The path once used becomes the path of choice. Herein lies the root of habit, and indeed of life itself; for were chance only to determine the path of the nerve current, no life, on our complex plane, would be possible. This, then, is our conception of the neuron pattern—a pathway formed, and inviting to subsequent travel. As regards its development and the cause of its persistence through the generations, it may be noted that the innate pattern is one which has "worked" in the past. Things done in a certain way, reactions of a certain kind, if successful and conducive to survival perpetuate themselves, for those who have such reactions *last best,* and have more children than those who react in some less useful manner. Of the thousands of possible reactions, by far the greater number, the poor ones, tend to die out—they do not work—and those who use them die out too. It is ever the successful useful pattern that survives and becomes the race tendency, though it may, too, of course, long outlive its period of usefulness.

It has been objected to this pattern conception that if a Chinese baby be brought up in England with English children it will behave as they do, and not as do the Chinese. But this signifies nothing—the major patterns with which we are chiefly concerned antedate all divergence of race and were undoubtedly common to the primitive ancestors of all. And as regards the minor differences in our inheritances, it must be remembered that a pattern is not believed to be a compelling control, but merely a *preferred* pathway—it does not function if the appropriate stimulus be lacking.

From the educational and developmental standpoint the pathways of especial importance are those laid down in the brain. The new-born babe has certain motor areas developed, and also certain perception areas—notably that of light vision, and, a little later, that of hearing—but these are all practically unconnected, and life begins on the simple reflex plan. The new-born babe takes in and gives out, but does not take in, turn over, and give out. As the days pass, however, these areas do gradually become connected, by what are called association fibres, until, soon, a stimulation received in one area is promptly passed on to the others, and the brain now begins to act as a whole. Thus, certain pictures produced in the visual, or auditory fields become associated with certain body sensations, as, for instance, with the discomfort of hunger, and, in turn, give rise to certain motor responses, such as the cry, and the extended hands.

It may be safely said that all life's development, all mental education, consists in adding to the associations possible, and in establishing those of most practical value to us. Pure sensation is possible only to the youngest infant—to all others sensation becomes a matter of appreciation, and is elaborated by associations until it attains to the appropriate response. Illustration seems superfluous, but to give just one—a gently turning door-knob makes no very frightful sound, but if you have supposed yourself to be alone in the house a door-knob so turning will not unlikely cause a cold chill of alarm. It is the association, of course, that arouses the response, and not at all the actual stimulus. The difference between the child and the adult, and between the feeble-minded and the normal, as well as between the beast and the man, lies in the relative perfection of their associations and in the elaboration of the pathways formed and available.

To reiterate, each of the pathways, whatever its elaboration of detail, constitutes a brain pattern, and if we go back to the thesis with which we began this chapter, it will be recognized that the innate disposition, there spoken of, is but an inherited *tendency* of pattern—a tendency to form certain brain patterns more easily than others. From ten thousand million cells an almost infinite variety of pattern is possible. Ten thousand million—just think what this figure means! It means, numerically, one cell for every six seconds of time since the first moment, of the first day, of year One of our era! But by physical inheritances in brain development, and in the spinal nerves as well, we obtain tendencies which lead the nerve force more aptly in certain directions than in others and make it more likely to be picked up by certain of the possible connecting cells. Why may a posthumous son stand and walk like his father? Why are some of us born Unitarians, and others of us Roman Catholics? The answers are obvious.

All the diversities of life trace back to the inherited, or acquired, brain pattern, and these, too, in their elaboration by association constitute the whole of psychology. Through all life the pattern remains, like a set-piece of fireworks, awaiting the spark—not always, of course, in consciousness, but ready always when the appropriate stimulus arrives.

In all this I have spoken only of the cerebro-spinal nerves, but it must be remembered that besides the cerebro-spinal system we have another, the sympathetic, and this, too, shares in the formation of the inherited patterns. It is this sympathetic system—a fine network of delicate nerve fibrils—which controls chiefly the involuntary actions, the blood vessels, the digestive, glandular and other organic functions; and it is to the activities of these sympathetic nerves, the oldest, in a developmental sense, of our bodies, that we owe our life process itself. It is from them, too, that we derive our emotions, for an emotion is but a sense appreciation by the brain of the action of the various glands and other organs.

Anatomically and physiologically the two systems of nerves are distinct, and yet they are connected—the sympathetic system having its origins in a series of nerve ganglia (groups of nerve cells) placed just in front of the spine, which ganglia directly connect with the cerebro-spinal system through the cord. So close is this connection that while the sympathetic nerves may, theoretically, be independently active, it is doubtful whether in man this ever actually occurs. It would seem, rather, that practically there is no operation of the one set of nerves without some reflected action of the other. A stimulus comes to us from without, is received by the cerebro-spinal nerves, is carried to the brain where it activates certain cells, and these, in turn, as we have already seen, send out currents over the motor nerves to the muscles. But part of this efferent force, also, it must be noted, flows through the connecting nerve filaments into the sympathetic system, and it is by this diverted current that the various glandular and other visceral changes are brought about. The "*affect*" of these organic changes, the sensation of them felt by the brain, is what we call an emotion; the immediate result of the changes—their *effect*—is a reinforcement of the action set up by the cerebrospinal system. Thus, a situation arises provocative of anger—the organic changes here seem due chiefly to sympathetic excitation of the adrenal glands—the blood pressure rises, the respiration is quickened, the heart beats more strongly and more rapidly, and the blood content is altered in the direction of providing an increase in elements conducive to muscle activity. In other words the body, sympathetically as well as consciously, prepares for increased self-expression—for fight.

Probably, as we have said, all mental experiences involve some stimulation of the sympathetic, but it is only when this stimulation becomes considerable that its effects rise into consciousness. The effects may there be entirely unregistered, or they may be sensed as mere "feeling," the result of a moderate stimulation; but again, this same stimulation, or another, sufficiently intensified, may rise to full consciousness with strong emotional value. *Interest* may be regarded as the mild pleasing affect associated with the motor state of attention and the innate disposition of curiosity; but with marked increase in intensity, with powerful stimulation, a true emotional state may develop.

We have, then, in the body two sets of nerves, the central or cerebro-spinal, and the visceral or sympathetic, these systems being independent, and yet related and connected to a degree that makes it possible, for all purposes of applied psychology, to treat of them as one. When a stimulus is received a nerve impulse darts here and there throughout the entire nervous system, and this impulse, or current, follows a path which has become preferred and established largely by the needs of our ancestors. Further, these inherited, preferred pathways of flow constitute for us the foundation of our innate dispositions. To understand our reactions fully, the sympathetic and cerebro-spinal systems must both be considered, but in this inheritance from the remote past it is the sympathetic, with the emotion it gives rise to, which is of first importance. As Bergson says: "We think with only a small part of our past, but it is with our entire past, including the original bent of our soul, that we desire, will, and act."

CHAPTER II

WITH the understanding of the nature of our inheritances as laid down in the first chapter, let us consider some of those which have a major importance both to man and to society. No exhaustive study can here be made, but let us get an idea of the psychological attitude in what must be but a paragraphic review.

We have found that physiologically the emotion is the result of gland action—a sensing of this action by the consciousness. Any stimulus may excite directly, or through some more or less realized idea, one or several of the glandular activities, and the glands so set in action will be those which by racial or individual experience have proven useful in similar situations. The sensing of the gland action, we say, constitutes the emotion. Now the sensations or affects most familiar to man have been dignified by names, but it must be evident that such naming is only a matter of convenience, that it can have no other significance. In fact the naming and classifying of the simple emotions, and the analysing of the more complex, is an exercise of ingenuity rather than of science.

In view of this fact it might be more truly scientific to effect our classification of the innate tendencies by reference to the instinctive purposes aimed at; but here at once we meet with the practical difficulty that there are too few such purposes to be useful for descriptive analysis. Going back in a search for the instinctive purpose, we find no ground to stand on until we arrive at those two primal urges —the striving, more or less consciously, toward self-preservation; and the striving, more or less unconsciously, toward the continuance of the race. A division into but two classes is not helpful, and yet, when we begin to further subdivide, when we begin to note the kinds and qualities of strivings, and the varied methods by which the instinctive longings are satisfied, then we find ourselves back on the emotional basis, and once again our classification becomes a matter of language. As usual, man reads his own ideas of "order" into the great complex of nature, but, as by so doing he makes it more comprehensible to his finite mind, the method can not yet be abandoned.

There is a tendency with laboratory psychologists to deny the primitive nature of many of the emotions now to be considered, but their judgment is largely based upon the study of the infant and is, therefore, inadequate. The infant has not the physiological and anatomic development of neurons necessary to reveal all of its instincts. Such development is to be obtained by growth only, and will arrive, in a normal child, as the need becomes established. But whether actually primitive or only "early conditioned," the significance of these reactions is the same, for they could not have been so uniformly developed throughout the race were they not the product of preferred, *i.e.* inherited patterns.

Fear

Fear is to be placed as one of the most primitive of man's emotional responses, and is common, too, to all but the lowest of animal life. Its purpose may be conceived as the preservation of the individual when faced by a superior and menacing power; and its expression, as the effort toward flight or concealment. With a child the full inheritance is here displayed, and here, more than with most inheritances, the primitive origin of our tendencies is revealed. That which was a menace to our earliest forest-living ancestors remains, today, a menace to the child. Sudden unfamiliar situations, loud and sudden noises, sounds which are harsh and gruff, low growling, and dark holes and corners, mysterious creakings, and creeping things—these are, with most, innately acknowledged as fearful, and innately call forth the appropriate response.

As reason develops, both emotion and expression become intellectually modified, but even in the adult the influence of the original tendency can generally be detected. The child reaction, being primitive, persists. "I expect in many growed-up men you'd call sensible there's a little boy sleepin'—the little kid they onced was—that still keeps his fear of the dark." * The fear of darkness may not be, strictly speaking, primitive, but darkness, with its uncertainties, has doubtless an aggravating effect on other fear-producing stimuli. The "tank," in the late war, was a creeping thing, and not a little to this fact was due its success as a demoralizing agent. The child is frightened by his playmate who has just donned a grotesque mask; and he laughs and he cries as his parent crawls toward him growling—reason and primitive emotion struggle for mastery, while already the emotion

* Owen Wister: *The Virginian.*

itself has become modified and softened until it
is almost a pleasure. In the highly complex
environment of modern life new elements and
dangers enter—these the child can have no
innate tendency to avoid—here reason alone
can determine the appropriate reaction, and the
child therefore approaches fearlessly that which
the parent regards with terror.

Here, then, is an example of all I have been
saying—an inherited emotional reaction following the brain and nerve patterns which have
been laid down in the experience of the past;
an emotion, with its accompanying motor expression, determining our present behaviour,
though modified now by added experience and
reason.

Physiologically, we find an excitation of the
adrenal glands, with increased body tensions,
and with general preparations for muscle activity. At least this is the case where the expression is to be that of flight. Where concealment
is the purpose very complex developments
occur; a degree of body tension is achieved, but
with it is a slowing of heart and respiration in
a general effort to avoid the slightest revealing
movement. Several glands are undoubtedly involved, and contrary tendencies develop—so in-
appropriately, at times, that the purpose of the

emotion becomes defeated. A paralysis of fear may be the outcome when flight is most urgently called for; and flight may inopportunely take place after safe concealment has been accomplished. Trembling is probably due to uncertain stimulation of opposing muscles, and may be brought about by the direct action of the adrenal secretion in the absence of control from the brain.

All this is from the individual standpoint. What part does this emotion play in social life?

Society, it has been stated, is an outgrowth from the needs of individual man. Though often jolted out of the normal evolutionary path by the revolutions of invention and discovery, it seems, however, to have been generally formed in response to man's emotional demands. The emotion of the individual passes into the social body and there determines the form of its institutions, but in this process remarkable transformations and strange developments occur.

Fear, for instance, while primitively useful, is nowadays, other than as caution and foresight, generally harmful. Nevertheless, fear is responsible for the foundation of that greatest of social forces, our religion. Let no one take offence. I refer to the elemental religion of primitive man, not to Christianity. The religion I write of is older than the New Testament—older, in fact, that the Old. Reverence, we shall find, is a compound of the primary emotions of wonder, negative self-feeling, tender emotion, and fear—having arrived at this fusion through the intermediate stages of admiration, awe, and gratitude. In other words, reverence is an elaboration possible only to a highly developed brain. The beginning of this complex, in primitive man, was fear.

Carlyle and others have attributed the birth of religion to awe and admiration. This concept is inspiring, but it is psychologically wrong, unless we begin our research at a period considerably later than that to which I refer. For primitive man did little wondering; he did not fall down in admiration of the rising sun, nor marvel at the broad expanse of the heavens —no more than does your child. These things he accepted as a matter of course. Had he been born in darkness, and had he reached maturity before these glories were revealed to him, then indeed he might have felt all that Carlyle has so beautifully portrayed. It was not the sun, the sky, the rain, that first caught man's attention, it was the lightning, the thunder, the flood, the tempest, and death. Here were destructive and malicious forces which did him harm. Before these he was powerless, and yet—after all, the lightning and thunder were only occasional, the flood was sometimes a useful stream, the rain was often a blessing, and death might threaten, and then withdraw. These forces were not, then, always malicious; their anger was sometimes abated. Is it not as with man? Let us propitiate these our enemies that they may harm us less often. Let us pay to them our devoirs.

Many centuries pass, and the nature forces, the *apseras*, the formless ones, become more and more anthropomorphic. Man is no longer, strictly speaking, primal, and religion is already becoming complex, but still the fear element prevails. Spirits of men and of supermen now live in the roar of the tempest. Man's ambitions and contests and jealousies are now seen in the alternations and contrasts of the natural phenomena. We are now at the period of our first contact with the Aryan beliefs—the Sky, the Sun, the Dawn are entering men's thoughts. Good gods appear, and struggle with the bad, but still the bad are the ones to be especially regarded—the good will do us no harm. Then, especially with those Aryans whose migrations had ended in gentle climes, the good gods begin to take precedence, and the evil of the old gods becomes but an angry mood of the new. But malicious god or angry good god, it is much the same—the fear *motif* remains as the chief determinant of worship. Fear now, too, becomes the basis of law and of morals. The propitiation of the gods becomes the tribal duty, and the individual who has done wrong, who has exposed the tribe to the wrath of the gods, is at once subjected to punishment. Magic, too, comes into play, and the priests, who once had only to instruct how harm might be avoided, are now consulted as a power in themselves, as having influence with the gods—an attitude not yet passed away.

For the next step our concern is with the Semitic belief. The tribal unity is broken, the priestly government is weakened, its subjects scattered, and the individual no longer fears the tribal revenge. How then shall justice be sustained? For man is now become a thinking animal and is asking questions. The wicked man prospers in this world? Evidently, then, he is to be punished elsewhere, so hell is invented. But this thinking man knows, too, that punishment long delayed is a poor deterrent from wickedness, so he offsets this fact, as well as he can, by making hell dreadful. The place

formerly of mere dark restlessness, endowed
with nothing worse than a social ennui, becomes
a place of eternal torment, under the control of
all the evil powers of the past, united now into
a sort of demon janitor—the devil. The Devil!
Who is he? He used to be called the Prince of
the Air—he was! He is the lineal descendant
of the old storm gods, exiled now, after being
stripped of all remnant of their occasional
virtue.*

This was long ago. Is fear no longer an
element in religion? The fact that many a
man today "experiences" religion only when
he is in trouble, or when he is near death,
may have some significance. Fear played
no part in the teachings of Christ, but how
about theology? How about the modern re-
vivalist? One recent particularly noisy ex-
ponent has based his entire system of salvation upon the old emotion of fear. In a
sense he is right, for if, as is claimed, intellectualism is killing religion, where is its injurious influence most felt? Is it not in its destruction of the belief in hell—in the removal of the
fear element from man's conception of the
results of his actions? "Take away the hope
of heaven—take away, much more, the fear of

* Keary: *Primitive Belief.*

31

hell, and you are going to be left with, at best,
an attitude of mere politeness toward the Com-
mandments.''* Man is still primitive, after
all; it is only the few who may safely shed the
old motive. And religion is not of the intellect;
it must always remain emotional.

Are we then, in our vanity, to sneer at the
past, and ourselves degenerate into a world of
atheists? Or, are we to recall a message which
was earnestly and lovingly preached, twenty
centuries ago, to the world's dull ears? Why
not turn back to that message, and to that
Teacher, and, in the tender emotion which
underlay all of His thoughts find now that impulse we so need toward Good? It is a long
way from the fearsome and malicious gods of
primitive man to the stern and jealous god of
Genesis; it is further from the god of Genesis
to the God of the Hebrews after the Captivity.
The next step, taught us so many centuries ago
by Christ, might now be ventured.

Anger

Fear is the safe response before superior
power—where there is equality, or where for
any reason there is a possibility of successful
self-assertion, the appropriate emotion, from

* Katherine Fullerton Gerould: *Atlantic Monthly, August,* 1920.

the primitive standpoint, is anger, with its motor expression, the fight.

We have here an assertion of self against interference from without; an assertion of the ego, which, to go back to the beginning, was probably once sexual—a defence of the mate, and an assertion of individual rights against the intrusion of interlopers. While fear goes back to our primitive ancestors, anger goes back at least as far, as is evidenced by its instinctive expressions. Hands, and nails (claws), and teeth are the weapons, as are, later, the club, and the convenient stone. The snarl and the sneer are common to dog and to man—they are but the display and threat of the "canine" teeth. The child claws and strikes and bites, using the weapons which nature long ago taught its forbears to use. Physiologically, in anger, as in fear, we have an excitation of the adrenal glands.

From primitive anger and its motor tendency toward fight, comes, later in the development of man, competition and emulation, business determination, and political and social strivings. In fact, in one sense, the disposition toward fight is but a form of efferent expression which may be aroused by any interference with our ego. It is the end product of any emotion the expression of which is strongly desired but prevented. It is the urge which carries us over our difficulties, and it is, therefore, of the utmost social interest.

This egotistic reaction has played a very large part in the growth of civilization, even in its primitive form. Our western world presents but a record of struggle, with the survival of the fittest, and law has become largely synonymous with force. Has the influence always been bad? Let us see. That in physical struggle the physically strongest may win is, of course, true, but physical strength, especially in group and national fights, is by no means alone in determining the result; physical strength often bows before social development and worth. Co-operation, foresight, and recognition of leadership are richly social attributes, and they are, too, factors which make for ultimate success in war. It is the strongest which wins, but the strength is to be measured by moral as well as by physical superiorities. The natural selection of war does not necessarily, nor often, lead to the perpetuation of mere brute force; it leads, rather, to the fixing of the more valuable social accomplishments. Those who lack these accomplishments lose out in the contest, and gradually disappear; those who have them most are victorious, and by their children perpetuate them.

That the late great war has apparently been destructive only, that no good at all can be seen as a result, is possibly due to our lack of perspective. However, despite many opinions to the contrary, it does not seem to me that the late war should be held responsible for the present world chaos—the war was but an incident, great as it was! Our social structure has long been growing top-heavy and menacing; it was already creaking, and splitting, and tottering when Germany threw in her bomb. The wreckage which has followed the explosion is no common result—it was precipitated by, but not due to the bomb.

Some of the effects of this founding of our western civilization on so strenuous an emotion are most interesting historically. Let me refer to one. Buddhism and Christianity are alike religions of peace, and both were born of peace-loving Asiatic races; but while the former found at once its natural habitat, and became a religion in fact—a religion which its professors were expected to practise—the latter met with a somewhat different fate, and its acceptance was long delayed. Buddhism stayed at home, but Christianity flowed westward, and, largely under the influence of the political power of Rome, was "handed" to Europe. What then is the situation? Here is a religion founded on love and peace, in a society founded on competition and fight. No wonder lip-service became the only service possible; no wonder there has remained so vast a discrepancy between the profession and the fact. Chesterton says that it is not that Christianity has been tried and found wanting, but that it has been found difficult, and so has not been tried. The peaceful Asiatic is true to his peaceful religion; the warlike European makes but a sorry adjustment to his.

In the sublimations of this same primitive emotion—in the intense striving of business, the modern version of the old fight instinct—the same differences are seen; the Asiatic remains passive and incapable when faced by his pugnacious western rival. Japan is no exception, it is a further endorsement of the idea, for Japan has Malay as well as Mongol ancestors, and the Malays fight. As a result, Japan treats its religion as an ethical ornament, as do we ours in the West; and Japan, also, maintains shops on Broadway. Leaving Japan aside, the East is the East and the West is the West, and the line of cleavage lies deep in the inherited tendencies of man.

CHAPTER III

OTHER INHERITED DISPOSITIONS, INCLUDING THE SEX
INSTINCT, TENDER EMOTION, AND PLAY

DISGUST is an expression of repulsion, and like
fear is an aversion, but here with the thought of
rejection of the offending object, rather than
with that of escape from it. Primitively, true to
the etymology of the word itself, it is associated
almost entirely with food, and it is still accompanied today, though now highly modified and
extended intellectually, with this same gastric
relation. We express nausea and disgust by the
same facial expression, and our language still
records the connection. That which disgusts us
"makes us sick," and inelegant man still spits
on the ground to show his lack of love for his
boss.

Positive and *negative self-feeling* are emotions of importance. The former reveals itself in
a tendency toward self-assertion, and is therefore closely related to anger; while the latter,
with its tendency toward self-abasement, is correspondingly related to fear. They might, indeed, be considered as intellectual derivatives

of these more primitive and grosser emotions, were it not that their presence is evident in animals other than man and it is still convenient to reserve the idea of intellectual refinement to the latter. *Bashfulness* is conceived of as an alternation of positive and negative self-feeling.

Curiosity, the tendency to approach and investigate, is also elemental in the same sense as above, namely, that it appears in many of the lower animals. Once a preservative tendency, asking, ''Is it dangerous?'', it has since become extended until now it is one of the roots of much of man's research, invention, discovery, and study. From asking ''Is it dangerous?'', it has now come to asking ''Will it work?'' *Wonder* is a fusion of curiosity with negative self-feeling, and is therefore not elemental.

The *gregarious instinct* has but a vague emotional content—a vague sense of lack, an intangible but real sense of uneasiness when one has become separated from one's kind. It is strong with certain animals urging them to strenuous endeavour to reunite with the herd. With man it varies greatly in strength, but the part it plays socially is a large one, it being a principal determinant in all man's foregathering, whether for social purposes, for sight-seeing, or for pleasure; and it is, too, one of the great factors in the huge growth of our cities. The same motive which originally brought animals together for safety is now a large part of, though not identical with, that which we call the "social instinct."

The Sex Instinct

In our opening remarks on the inherited dispositions we found that if these be studied from the standpoint of their purpose all fall into one or other of two categories—those looking toward self-preservation, and those which tend to perpetuate the race. The dispositions of the first class are real and personal, and conscious of their end; those of the second are equally real and personal, but are largely unconscious of end. In this second class the sex instinct is paramount.

According to Freud, sex feeling is at the root of all life, and it is the sex impulse, the "libido," which supplies all our energy, whether in sex relations or in matters intellectually far removed from sex. Freud has made a valuable contribution to psychology in propounding this idea, and yet such use of the term *sex* would seem rather unfortunate. The word has a distinct connotation in our minds, and, for the great vital urge, a more general term would seem advisable—some such term as Bergson offers in his "*élan vital.*" This last, be it understood, is directly comparable with Freud's "libido," the impulse of life itself; but, with Bergson the sex desire becomes merely one of the manifestations of this impulse—to me a more useful conception.

As regards sex problems, whatever opinion we may hold of their nature, however important they may be in sociology, pathology, and criminology, however large a part they may play in our happiness and our miseries, we may still erect a fairly complete system of psychology without them. They are concrete and largely social. Such reference as we have to make to them will be in our consideration of the mental ills. In the sex instinct itself, however, we approach more nearly to the true animal instinct than we do in any other of man's inheritances, and for this reason it is well worth discussion here. It should lead us to a clearer conception of instinct in general.

Regard for a moment the marvels of instinctive action in the life of the insect. When the mud wasp squeezes the head of the caterpillar, and benumbs it, and then proceeds to puncture successively its nine principal nerve centres, it does this with no intellectual understanding of the caterpillar's anatomy. When the nectar-loving insect plants its eggs in a bit of carrion, it does this with no understanding of the future food needs of the larvae. When the beetle *Sitaris* places its eggs so that they shall ultimately be carried to their best habitat, it does this with no knowledge of the long series of steps they must traverse. Just so long as we retain any thought of finding intellectual acts here hidden, just so long do we continue in an incomprehensible world of mystery. If, as Bergson says, the consciousness which lurks in instinct could be awakened to knowledge it would touch the most intimate secrets of life.

Let the *why* remain a mystery—the *how*, even, is not known. But as to the *how* let me venture a flight of imagination. Stimuli come to the body, so far as we know, only through the receptive end-organs of the cerebro-spinal nerves, but it is conceivable that appreciations may come, also, directly through the sympathetic system. It is by these sympathetically received appreciations that I would, tentatively, explain the instinct of animals. And, be it noted, in the hymenoptera, where instinct is truly triumphant, there is no cerebro-spinal system existing. Instinct is feeling, not reasoning—the broody hen does not plan a family, but, as James says, regards her nestful of eggs as an "utterly fascinating and precious, and never-to-be-too-much-sat-upon object." I am sure that when the brood hatches, at least the first brood, mother hen is often sore puzzled.

Apply this to sex. It is common with psychologists to speak of an "instinct of reproduction," but how can such an instinct be? Reproduction is an intellectual concept—not instinctive. The sex impulse, it seems to me, sweeps away all *ideas;* it is a *feeling,* a most intense one, and reproduction is but a result of its satisfaction. The insect does things of vital importance to the continuance of its species, but it does them with no idea of that end—it does them to satisfy a desire, and so does man. The sex instinct, like all true instincts, is a compelling desire, not an intellectual concept evolving the idea of reproduction. As a matter of fact, when the idea of reproduction does enter the mind it may act as a deterrent and check.

Here, then, in the true instinct of sex, is a powerful urge, an emotional wave, which, satisfied, starts in operation a sequence of events resulting nine months later in a baby! Is there any more wonderful phenomenon in nature than this? Does the insect accomplish any more marvellous feat in the finding of the appropriate home for its eggs? Primitive man knew no more of biology than does the lowest animal today, and few among men now deliberately seek the intellectually appreciated end of their act.

I hold, then, that the instinct is of sexual desire, and not of reproduction; and that it is by our knowledge of this desire that we are led to an understanding of the animal instinct.

Intellectualization of this sex instinct has produced some curious results. So far are the extremities of the sexual function separated in man's mind, that the first step, its inception, has always been counted as more or less shameful, and the last step, its culmination, has been esteemed as a blessing. Gods and heroes have been gloriously born into this world, but so firmly is the idea of an unworthy carnal lust attached to the beginning of the great miracle of nature, that theologians, and peoples, have always felt it necessary to provide for them a supernatural or immaculate conception.

The sexual instinct is at the root of all society. By it man and woman were brought together, and by it the family came. With the family came the discovery of the advantage of division of labour; came, too, adjustment and self-sacrifice—a sense of duty to the group, and the principle of submergence of personal rights in the face of the public (family) need.

Tender Emotion

Tender emotion, the parental instinct, is that altruistic impulse which leads to the protection of the young, and is strongest in those animals whose young require protection the longest. It is at the foundation of all unselfishness and is, therefore, of eminent importance in the social group.

In the primitive concrete expression, tender emotion is characteristically a female instinct, and might be called the maternal, but it varies greatly in strength in different individuals. One little girl loves her doll devotedly and tenderly cares for it; another leaves her doll out in the rain. One mother lives a life of sacrifice for her children, and another finds her instinct fully satisfied by turning her children over to the servants. Throughout woman's life, the instinct, if it exists at all, commonly preserves its primitive form, and its connection with childhood remains easily traceable. Woman's affections and interests incline to the *little*

44

things, to helpless things, and she speaks of
"the dearest little house," "the cutest little
box," "the darlingest little boat," and even of
"dear little Belgium." Note, too, the language
of endearment in the mushy stage of love, when
some husky brute is fondled as "Baby"!

With man the parental instinct is probably
less strong than with woman, and what passes
for it is often a complex emotion in which
egotism is no slight component. In its exten-
sions, too, man tends to the abstract. Little
things do not appeal so strongly as do general
principles of justice. The sense of equity and
justice are psychologically male possessions, involving abstract judgments, which in women
are obstructed by the concrete personal appeal.

We have mentioned "dear little Belgium."
Since 1914 this expression has become charged
with a compound emotional value, and anger
uniting itself with tender emotion has produced
what we call *moral indignation*.

Often confused with tender emotion is—*sympathy* (a suffering with), the tendency to take
to one's self the suffering of another, or, better,
the emotional state of another. The contemplation of the emotion of another excites into activity corresponding nerve patterns within our-

selves. The emotion so transferred is not always painful; one dog barks, one man yawns, one member of a herd becomes excited, and—all dogs within hearing bark, the man's vis-à-vis yawns, and the herd stampedes. Even a pretence of emotion will start a similar reaction in one who is especially sympathetic—as witness the contagious laugh, the tears in the theatre, and the distress of a child when its mother pretends to cry.

Note that this is very different from tender emotion. Sympathy may lack all altruistic feeling and may be strong in an absolutely self-centred person. The tendency of sympathy itself, alone, is to get away from the sight and hearing of suffering. A man who is made miserable by a recital of pain may not lift his hand to relieve it. It was a sympathetic man who said that he could not bear to see women standing in the trolley car—so always pretended to be asleep.

When sympathy combines with tender emotion, then we have a truly useful compound, that which we know as *pity*. Here the pain of sympathy is sweetened by the altruistic impulse. The Priest and the Levite may both have had sympathy, but the Good Samaritan was moved by pity.

OTHER INHERITED DISPOSITIONS

In the tender emotion, the elements of our Christian religion are to be found. Christ's message was based upon the tender emotion; it was the conception of a loving Father that he gave to the world. Trust and gentleness were to replace fear and anger, and brotherly love the strivings of egotism.

Play

We come now to a tendency which differs from all that have preceded, in that it has, in itself, no specific emotional content. I refer to play.* The play tendency in the child and in other young animals has been generally explained from the standpoint of purpose, as a preparation for adult life—a strengthening of muscles and a developing of useful co-ordinated movements. Now young animals certainly do imitate in their play the actions which will be useful to them later on, but purposeful acts no longer occupy the position they once did in psychological thought. Nature is no longer conceived of as always looking ahead—this prophetic spirit is now denied her. The fact is that play must be explained on a very different basis, though the results may truly be as useful as stated.

* Compare G. T. W. Patrick: *The Psychology of Relaxation.*

In the development of life certain primitive brain patterns become far more deeply graven than do others. These patterns are the earliest, the most used, and, in individual growth, the first brought to maturity; they are, too, the *easiest,* for dog and for puppy, for man and for child. Herbivorous animals *run* in play—even the non-humorous lamb manages to skip about a bit. Hunting animals play at *fighting.* One puppy rolls another and grabs him by the throat; the kitten crouches, creeps, and then springs on the spool. Here we have, truly, apparently a prevision of what is to come, but it is really only a looking backward, a response to the early formed, and therefore early matured, brain and nerve patterns just mentioned. We might beg the question and say that play reveals the primitive and must be studied to know the primitive. It is as with the psychology of the crowd, to be later considered, it opens a window through which we may view the past.

The child, in his play, does not do things of especial use to him in his future life—except, of course, in the way of general muscle development—he reverts to primitive memories. Early man lived in the forest and fought with wild beasts, and he did this for hundreds of thousands of years—he has become civilized only

48

since yesterday. The strongly set patterns with which he now starts life are those of the long forest period. The boy runs, wrestles, climbs, throws stones, and wields clubs, and, when he gets older, he hunts and he fishes. He did these things back in the days when most of Europe was still buried under ice; or, if he did not, he died very young and therefore left no non-running, non-hitting, non-striking children to succeed him.

It is the *motor* tendencies that are first developed, and which are revealed in play; the full emotion of the original action for which they stand has yet to come. The so-called restraint of play is but a negative phenomenon—it is the absence of a desire to hurt, with, possibly, a subconscious sense that if one does hurt one will then suffer isolation. However, play becoming very intense may easily develop the emotion originally lacking—the play of dogs and of boys often ends in a fight.

I have referred only to the play of the boy-child. As regards his sister, there is this difference, that while both boy and girl follow the oldest race patterns, the antiquity of their patterns is not equally evident. With the boy their primitive nature is recognizable from the fact that as he grows, in this present social world, he

49

is compelled to abandon them, or to reserve them for selected occasions; while with the girl these old patterns are, today, as useful as ever —though she is trying to think otherwise. Old as they are, the patterns of womanhood are still ever modern, and still remain socially the best. The dearly beloved doll so sweetly nursed is but the surrogate for the child-to-be. I believe truly that the future welfare of the race depends upon the doll-loving little girl of today. We may add, however, for the solace of those who do not care for dolls, that the maternal instinct, the tender emotion of maternity, is sometimes late in developing, and may even not come until the arrival of the first real baby.

But to return to play considered as the operation of easy old patterns. With this conception of its origin, the play of the adult is equally explained. Man tires by too long application to social and business affairs, and needs rest. The modern achievements demand the exercise of the more recently developed brain areas and these, precisely because they are so recent, fatigue the more quickly. Even "being good" too long may become burdensome; the too close application of the modern moral conventions will wear. After a week at Chautauqua Professor James said he felt ready for any deviltry that might present. What does man do for the rest which he craves? He turns back to the older and simpler patterns. It is like taking off a tight pair of new shoes and putting on again the comfortable old ones. He goes to the woods; he lives in a tent; he wears old clothes; he hunts and he fishes; or he digs in the ground in the garden.

In speaking of the play of the adult, I am referring to the adult mind—something by no means always found in the grown-up body. Extravagant devotion to play and perpetual seeking for entertainment belong to the child mind, and, when found in the adult, are, in themselves, evidence of the failure to grow up. It has been said that play is the business of the child, while it is man's relaxation, but to these grown-ups with childish minds play remains always a business. They need stimulation, not relaxation, and they seek this in shallow artificial amusements.

It is important to note that this reversion to earlier type in the adult, this relaxation of the spirit by return to the more elemental life, does not always take the innocent form of what we call play. Suppose one has never had a chance to play. Suppose one has been driven from morning to night with the demand for *efficiency*.

Suppose all natural expressions of relaxation and freedom are *verboten*. Then we may have war! The Germans did not play, but they reverted all the same, and they, too, took a vacation from the strenuous life by once more becoming elemental. The militaristic group, maybe, started it, but it was the German people who made it a national war, so eager were they to escape their fatigue. They reverted, and their reversion brought them to—what we have seen. It may be objected that war itself is far more wearing than that from which they were endeavouring to escape, but this is not the point. War is more primitive, and it is the primitive that we crave. Man hunts for wild game, and suffers all manner of hardships and dangers, but he returns to the wilderness each year, if he can but get away from his office. It is not a question of the suffering which may ultimately be realized; it is the call of the wild which must be responded to whatever the cost. What of the United States? We did not wish to fight, and yet we have been counted as passing strenuous, too. But we are a play-people, and already have more relaxation than we know what to do with.

One hears, today, the pre-war German decried as a hypocrite. That gentle friend who made your life so pleasant in your Berlin days was no hypocrite. He was sincerely your friend. What happened when he became ill—when he broke with the strain, and reverted—was quite as unexpected by him as by you.

CHAPTER IV

THE COMPOUND EMOTIONS, SENTIMENTS, TEMPERA-MENT, AND CHARACTER

The Compound Emotions

I HAVE mentioned *pity* as a compound of tender emotion and sympathy; and *moral indignation,* as a compound of tender emotion and anger. These are examples of compound emotions— emotions which become possible with the higher development of the brain. A fusion of impulses is here implied, and for this fusion the association areas of the brain must be highly developed. The possibility of forming such compounds is generally and necessarily lacking in early childhood, as it is almost invariably, also, in the feeble-minded and in animals. The weak-minded mother *alternates* her emotions, she can not fuse them; she beats her child viciously one moment, and hugs it affectionately the next. This a matter which must be kept always in mind in our dealings with children and with the feeble-minded, and—dare I add?—with the masses. From them we must be content to receive simple responses; we must not expect the more elaborate complexes possible to the highly developed.

Here, in this process of emotion compounding, lie all the finer variations in character. Pity is a compound of tender emotion and sympathy, but in two persons, and in a thousand, it may vary in value, changing always with both the actual and relative amounts of its component parts.

Hate, so far as it can be considered a compound emotion, may be regarded as a composite of anger, disgust, and fear; or, possibly, instead of the last named, a negative self-feeling. But hate is, too, and more properly, classed as a sentiment, and will be later considered. Disgust unites with positive-feeling, and the compound so formed, when exhibited before an equal or a superior, we call *Scorn;* whereas the same compound directed against an inferior is termed *Contempt.* Disgust and fear produce *Horror* or *Loathing.*

Wonder, negative self-feeling, and fear, give us *Awe;* negative self-feeling and tender emotion are important elements in *Gratitude;* while awe and gratitude unite in the emotion of *Reverence.*

Sorrow may be regarded as a painfully toned

compound of frustrated tender emotion with negative self-feeling. *Grief* has an element of resentment and combined with the frustrated tender emotion, we find instead of a negative self-feeling as in sorrow, a frustrated positive self-feeling. *Regret* is a looking to the past; either a frustrated desire or a reaction from a desire which has been yielded to; while *Remorse* is a regret plus anger—an anger which, being directed against self, becomes particularly painful as it can find no relief in expression. It being the self-regard which is wounded, even penance can not satisfy. *Reproach* is a modified moral indignation, consisting, as does the latter, of a fusion of anger and tender emotion. In reproach, the two emotions are aroused by the same object; whereas in moral indignation, the tender emotion is directed toward one, while the anger is directed toward another who threatens that one. *Anxiety* may be regarded as an anticipatory pain combined with tender emotion. *Revenge* arises from a fusion of anger and wounded positive self-feeling; or, it may be considered as anger restrained by calculation. *Jealousy* is the painful feeling resulting from lack of reciprocation—it is an emotion of a frustrated sentiment of love where the positive self-feeling, egotism, has been a principal component. In it we find the elements of anxiety, revenge, and reproach.

Bashfulness I have referred to as an alternation of positive and negative self-feeling, and it is not, therefore, a compound at all; but *Shame* is an emotional state related to remorse. *Modesty, Courage, Generosity,* and *Meanness* are character attributes developed with and within the sentiments.

In this analysis of the compound emotions I have followed, largely, McDougall and Ribot, but it must be remembered, as has been already remarked, that this classifying of the emotions is a matter of convenience only and, strictly speaking, one of language; one must not take it too seriously. The glandular and other visceral origins of these mental affects, which it has pleased us to name, will in themselves permit of no such arbitrary delimitation. The body acts and reacts as a whole, and its flowing waves of energy recognize no man-made classification —nature does not lend itself to this sort of thing. What is important, here, is to recognize that from the same elemental reactions which are common to man and beast there has grown, by the development of areas of association within the brain, all the highly complex emotional possibilities we now know.

Sentiments

We have passed from simple reflexes to the simple emotional reactions, and from these, with the increasing powers of association, to the compound emotions. The next step in character formation is in the development of the sentiments.*

A sentiment may be defined as an organized system of emotional dispositions centred about the idea of some object. Or, it may be defined as an idea with emotional associations and, therefore, with emotional values and potentialities. In the latter sense it is but an elaboration of the primary and compound emotions already considered—the result of association—differing only in the strength of the central idea, and in the number of emotional tendencies which may be stimulated by it. What is an idea? Is it not itself the product of elaboration? From reflex nerve actions which may or may not reach consciousness, we pass to those which do produce in the brain a characteristic sensory affect. By further development a brain pattern is formed, a sensory memory results, and this, by association, becomes linked with other memories until a system is developed. In

* Compare Professor McDougall's *Social Psychology*.

this system, once formed, the central pattern may be aroused into activity apparently without external stimulation. An idea comes to us seemingly without reference to any external impression, but the impression has been there, nevertheless; it has come to us through one of the associated areas. Thus it is, too, that an idea may become stronger in memory than it was in its original production, an increased emotional value having been obtained by the associations which are subsequently made. See how the memory of an insult grows.·

Our conception of the sentiment differs from that of the idea only in our orientation toward it. The sentiment we find in the complex as a whole, existing as a central dominant idea with numerous emotional associations ready to be awakened, in turn, as occasion demands. Let us illustrate. Love and hate are typical sentiments. Here a complex of emotional associations, a system, is erected around the idea of some individual, making everything that pertains to that individual of emotional value. Thus, you love a person, and you experience tender emotion in his presence, anxiety when he is in danger, anger when he is criticized, joy when he prospers, and sorrow when he dies.

Or, consider the building of a sentiment. A child has a violent tempered father, always scolding and punishing. At first, the child experiences fear at each exhibition of bad temper, and then only, but gradually the fear comes to be aroused by the mere presence of the father—a habit of fear has been formed—and, finally, the thought of the father is sufficient. This we may call a sentiment of fear, with the father as the central idea. As the child grows older, and new associations are made, it comes to experience, in addition to the fear, anger, disgust, and resentment. The child has now acquired a sentiment of hate.

It is interesting to note that a sentiment will determine the value of all experiences which come to us in association with it. A girl "hates" a dress in which she has once been a wall-flower. We dislike a person—he utters some opinion—instantly we dislike that opinion. We like a person—he utters the same opinion—we are at once all interest and receptive attention.

We are, in fact, largely ruled by our sentiments, and therefore it is that when one limited sentiment becomes dominant in our lives, as it may, our judgments cease to be valuable. So it is that enthusiasts, fanatics, and all one-idea people are worthless as counsellors. When David Copperfield fell in love with Dora, Dora became the central idea about which he ranged all his emotions. A dominant Dora sentiment came into existence. He lived, breathed, dreamed, and ate Dora. The minister preached, and it was about Dora. At his work in the Commons, it was Dora, not the judge, who presided. He was steeped in Dora, saturated through and through with Dora. "Enough love," he says, "might have been wrung out of me, metaphorically speaking, to drown everybody in; and yet there would have remained enough within me and all over me, to pervade my whole existence." And Dora, we know, was but a feeble-minded child!

From these extreme experiences in mortal love—alas!—there is generally an awakening. With the satisfaction of the senses there is a gradual disintegration of the sentimental complex; older associations come back into play, and judgment of value again finally asserts itself. On the other hand, with love that is worthily placed, and, also, with love that can not attain to its object (with mortal love sometimes, but more frequently with devotion to the unattainable divine) the sentiment may become permanent and remain the dominant control

61

throughout life. Witness the lives of the saints.

As we know, all sentiments are not, unfortunately, so pleasant as is that of love. Where fear and anger enter in, the sentiment is both unpleasant and harmful. If a sentiment of this type obtain control, the results are often serious both to health and to one's social enjoyments. The boy who has acquired a sentiment of hate for his father may extend this to include all those who resemble his father, and then to all men, and, finally, to all people. The end result is a misanthrope, or a recluse.

The sentiments, it will be noted, are all emotionally induced; they are complexes of emotions, and are, therefore, unreasonable things which may operate, as we have seen, either for good or for bad. *Happiness consists in having only well-ordered, non-conflicting, perfectly compatible sentiments, from which the destructive emotions of fear and anger have been eliminated.* Joy and happiness may be regarded as the mental sensing of this smooth harmonious brain action, just as *pleasure* is that which is felt in the physiological gratification of the minor impulses.

Intellectually, of course, we may have a certain degree of control over our sentiments, and we speak of a "well-balanced person," meaning, generally, one so endowed. But life's problems are many, and, to the acute observations of the highly cultivated man, life's experiences are no simple thing to adjust. Compromise only is possible—compromise and intellectual command. Hence it is that happiness, light-hearted happiness, is rare in the world's great men. This is a state which can be attained by them, it would seem, only after a retrograde process, a process of elimination—a conversion, which is really a reversion. Here is a going back to child-like simplicity—"of such only is the Kingdom of Heaven." In this process of conversion a man who has gradually erected a religious sentiment suddenly awakens to a realization that this sentiment has become large enough for him to live entirely within. He then rejects the past and the old, forsakes all his former external, conflicting associations, substitutes trust for fear, and eliminates anger, and from now on leads a new, more limited, but entirely harmonious and, therefore, happy life.

The greatest happiness is, as has been said, when *all* the sentiments are in harmonious relation, but a degree of happiness is possible, too, when dominant sentiments only have been so correlated—when the things we most care about have been erected into a harmonious whole. This being accomplished we can well afford to ignore the lesser experiences should these become annoying. A mind so ordered, when real losses do come, experiences sorrow rather than grief—and then it is that the less endowed of us wonder at the beauty of their quiet resignation. What with us would give rise to grief and resentment, with them, having no anger nor fear in their hearts, arouses no evil conflict at all. Here is the happiness of simpleminded strongly religious people. To these well unified personalities, with their gentler emotions all oriented into one dominant whole, with fear and anger excluded, distresses may come—pain, martyrdom even, but, entering into their beatified sentiment toward God, these evil things lose all of their force.

In regard to the valuation of sentiments, we must remember, as with the emotions in general, that all is not said when a name has been given, nor even, in these complex systems of emotions, when we specify their component parts. The value is dependent rather upon the proportionate amounts of these parts, and upon their relative strengths. Thus an infinite variation in value is possible for each and every sentiment of man. For instance, positive self-feeling, desirably present in many sentiments, may in some, by becoming unduly prominent, take away all social worth. In love, for example, a strong egotistic emotion, revealing itself in pride of possession, in gratified ownership, as well as in jealousy, may rob the sentiment of all of its beauty. Here we have the father who loves his son so long as he can take pride in the son's accomplishments, but who becomes impatient and intolerant at failure. As we have it in Proverbs, "The father of a fool hath no joy." The mother, with her stronger strain of tender emotion, cares little for the boy's failures; indeed she rather inclines to the weakling as more needing her care.

I say the emotion of positive self-feeling may rob a sentiment of all social value, and yet, among the more conspicuously useful sentiments we have that of *self-regard,* a sentiment actually built round *self* as the central idea. Here we have a sentiment which in its simplest form is purely selfish, but which has been extended in one way or another until it has mounted to the highest reaches of altruism. The idea of self has enlarged until it has embraced the family, the home, the group, and the nation, and, finally, the whole of mankind.

Within this sentiment, then, there is a long range of values depending on its form and development. Here we find the individual egotist, the family man, the patriot, and the philanthropist. And, again, the values vary with the persistence with which the original egotism survives through these steps of altruistic growth. With strong egotism the family man may be simply a man who is inordinately vain of his family; the patriot may be that useless and dangerous citizen who sees nothing but good in his own country, and nothing but bad in others; and the philanthropist may be one whose incentive is, secretly, a love of popular approval.

The sentiment, then, is highly complex and for its formation, as has already been said, a very considerable brain development is essential. In the child and in the feeble-minded, with their slight powers of association, there can be but few and very imperfect sentiments; as there can be, also, as we have already seen, but few even of the compound emotions. The child and the imbecile are constantly changing their attitudes—miserable one moment and happy the next, responding always to what the present may offer. Instead of fusions and well oriented systems we find only alternations of the simple emotions. Bear this fact in mind and you will not be surprised at the crude reactions one so frequently meets with in inferior mentalities. Goddard tells of a murderer who was more concerned over a debt of sixty cents which was owing him, than he was over his impending punishment. He tells, too, of a feeble-minded woman who after relating the recent loss of her three children, all within a period of two weeks, added, "That's going some, ain't it?"

This "callous" criminal and this "cold-hearted" mother are simply examples of individuals whose brains have not developed to the degree where elaborate associations and sentiments have become possible. With this mother there was no *sentiment* of love, and hence no possibility of sorrow. Tender emotion there may have been, but for the exhibition of this the children must actually have been present. With the criminal, in the case cited, there was the same lack of sentiment formation, the same child-like absorption in the present—but the criminality itself, of course, is not to be taken as any evidence of deficiency. Again, sentiments may exist but they may be bad ones. There are those of whom it has been said that, like the crab, having made sure they are right, they go ahead for all they are worth—sideways. With the man—not the crab—faulty education and bad environment are here generally responsible.

I have mentioned only love, hate, the religious sentiment, and the self-regarding sentiment, but sentiments may be built within any of the spheres of life's activities—in science, music, art, and studies; in the acquisition of wealth and position, in business, and in the social world. Whatever the field the process is the same. We advance from the primary emotion to the compound, and from this to the sentiment, all by the forming of more and more brain patterns, more and more associations, and, then, by gradually orienting these into homogeneous groups. Out of the complexity and confusion of life we thus again approach order and harmony by regimenting our thousands of experiences into one or more systems, each gathered around some central idea.

Temperament

The innate dispositions so far mentioned are those dependent upon brain association and, ultimately, upon the possession of definite brain patterns. One other inheritance we have, and this is our temperament. Here we are concerned, not with patterns, but with the general health and vitality of the body, and, especially, with the condition of the nerves, the nerve cells and the glands. The temperament, then, may be thought of as the soil in which the pathways of disposition are laid down.

Back in the second century, Galen wrote of the four humours of the body—the blood, the phlegm, the yellow bile, and the black. Our language still perpetuates Galen, and we now speak of the sanguine, the phlegmatic, the choleric, and the melancholic—the warm-blooded, the dull, the irritable, and the sentimentally sad.

Here we have mankind divided into groups, characteristic and isolated, in that they have no mutual understanding. From all time the sanguine have been hitting the phlegmatic on the back, and telling them to wake up. The choleric tell the sanguine that they are altogether too amiable, and, in their hearts, think them shallow and frivolous. The phlegmatic wish the others would leave them alone; and all together unite in an effort to cheer up the melancholic. No, not all! The phlegmatic don't care. And so it is, each group regards the others with mixed feelings, but in these there is always a something of criticism.

Transient temperamental changes may be produced by transient physical conditions. Illness may alter the whole mental atmosphere; as witness the choleric and melancholic states set up by the liver. That whether life is worth living depends on the liver, is often profoundly true. Melancholy, the black bile of the ancients, is often a liver disease, and may exhibit itself in all degrees of dejection down to absolute hopelessness and suicide.

Character

Let us sum up all that has gone before, and arrive at a definition of character.

The disposition, we have found, is the sum of our innate tendencies. The temperament is the result of our nervous, glandular, and other organic vitalities. *The character is the sum of the innate dispositions, plus the physiologically determined temperament, plus the sum of all the acquired tendencies.* It is the product of the interaction of the disposition and temperament with the environment.

Here at last we have something which seems in some degree modifiable. With the two inherited factors we have now one that is acquired, and which, we shall find, leads us away from the emotions, and into the intellectual field. We go back to a consideration of brain patterns, but principally now to those which we make for ourselves.

CHAPTER V

IT was said, when first speaking of brain patterns, that a nerve force flowing over a certain path produces some change in the nerve cells which renders that path more easily traversed by a subsequent current. In this lies the beginning of a habit. It is the brain pattern, once more, viewed now from but a slightly different angle. Suppose the nerve current again and again to traverse the same path—it flows with greater and greater ease, it cuts, as it were, a deeper and deeper channel, until, what probably in the beginning required a deliberate and conscious effort, comes, finally, to be performed automatically. Suppose a certain action involves a series of steps, A, B, C, D, E, F—the first time this act was performed each step involved thought and decision, but with each repetition the effort becomes less until, finally, the steps are taken quite unconsciously. All that is necessary from now on is to set A going—B naturally follows, then C, and so on to the completion at F.

As one need hardly remark, habit formation is of great importance in life; so important, in fact, that life can not well be conceived of without it. Walking, eating, and dressing, and speech itself are habit processes—which, fortunately for us, we do not easily depart from nor forget. When we do, when through brain disturbances these early formed paths become obliterated, the life of the patient is a veritable misery. These are essential habits, but in all of our waking day habits of one kind or another play a large part in making our lives both easy and possible. Our movements become both facile and automatic, and our attention, being thus released from the necessity of their detailed control, is free to turn itself elsewhere. Conscious attention to any detail is fatiguing— become conscious of the mechanism of walking, and see how far you can go! The principal cause of the fatigue of neurasthenia is simply that in this disease all acts become more or less conscious and have to be thought out.

Habits, then, simplify life. They help, also, in many other ways. We know, for instance, that certain acts are easy enough at certain times, but are performed unwillingly at others; it is then that habit steps in to make them more possible. It is largely habit that carries a woman through her housework when fatigued. It is often habit that takes a man to his office when he would rather stay at home. It is habit that preserves discipline and co-ordinated movement in the soldier during the stress of battle; and it was to form this so requisite habit that the long months of drill were necessary.

Habit training constitutes the very essence of education. When one considers that even one passage of the nerve force over a certain pathway tends to make that pathway more easily traversed a second time, giving it an advantage over all other pathways, it becomes evident that habit formation belongs properly to the period of childhood. If a child be permitted to grow up forming its nerve pathways by accident and by impulse, it will be ever at a disadvantage, for the bad habits so formed will probably persist throughout life. James says: "Could the young but realize how soon they will become a walking bundle of habits, they would give more heed to their conduct while in the plastic state." Alas! If youth but would, or if age but could! Since the child will not so realize, the duty of the parents becomes clear. What a fatal attitude it is to constantly excuse bad habits with, "He is only a child," as though when he grew older the habit could easily be broken! Some one has said that a habit "is a sort of gimlet; every year gives it another turn. To pull it out the first year is like plucking out the hair by the roots; in the second year, like tearing the skin; in the third, like breaking the bones; and in the fourth, like removing the very brain itself."

What are some of the elements in deliberate habit formation? Give full attention to the act, making as deep an impression as is possible upon the nerve cells; truly desire, truly want to do the thing right; then *act at once* and repeat regularly. Make, thus, a close association between the act and the intention, and *repeat even when inconvenient.* On the other hand, habits are deliberately broken by analyzing them and bringing their successive steps back into consciousness; and then, by focusing the attention upon the earlier steps and establishing for these new inhibitions and associations. Thus, in the habitual act involving steps *A, B, C, D, E,* and *F,* focus the attention on *A,* or *B,* inhibit these beginnings, or establish for them a new association in the mind. Let *A* now come habitually to suggest *X,* not *B,* thus diverting the current at its inception into an entirely new path. The new association, *X,* may be anything you please, anything you may find practically useful—the thought of a sacrifice with which you may have penalized yourself should you yield to the original impulse (James tells of a man who broke a saloon habit by offering fifty dollars to any one who should see him in a saloon), or, it may be, a prayer, or a promise to one's mother, or to one's own personal honour; or merely some diverting physical interruption, such as a walking round the room, or the square. Whatever you do, remember that when you content yourself with saying that you "won't count this time" you are, thereby, beginning the worst habit of all, namely, that of disregarding your good resolutions.

Socially, habit forms the basis of much of our more conservative behaviour. By it change is resisted and institutions perpetuated. It has, however, many vagaries as regards usefulness. In its persisting tendency it may long survive its original purpose, and what was once a good habit may become in the course of time either indifferent or harmful. Here we find the explanation of much of our ceremony, and here, too, both in ceremony and elsewhere, is the tendency to confuse the means with the end. An act begins, for instance, as a symbol of worship; it ends by itself becoming the one important fact. A man starts out to save money to provide for his old age, but the saving never ceases and the man slaves until his death. The housewife cleans her home that it may be more attractive and comfortable, but she never stops cleaning, and comfort departs.

Books have been written on this subject which I am treating so casually. I know of none other more important to comfort, to happiness, and to usefulness in life. Dallas Lore Sharp has said that we come to college with all of our educational clothing on, and that the college faculty just buttons it up and adjusts it. Let us paraphrase Professor Sharp—habit is clothing, as the word suggests—is it not equally true that we enter manhood with all of our habits on, and spend the rest of life trying to adjust them?

All of this, as I have said, is a matter of the brain pattern, and, in one sense, has a relation to instinct, using the latter term in the popular, loose way. Habit has been defined as an acquired instinct, and instinct, as an inherited habit—if we replace *instinct*, here, by *disposition*, then the statement may well be allowed to stand. The inherited disposition is an inherited brain pattern, or at least a potential pattern, one especially apt of development. The habit is the pattern, either acquired or inherited, made real and effective by use.

CHAPTER VI

MEMORY

ONCE more we examine the brain pattern, but now from the standpoint of the mental *record*, rather than from that of the *act* it leads to, the habit. As this last, the habit, was found to be at the root of all life's performances, so memory is the foundation of all mental processes. Furthermore, while it is convenient to distinguish between the mental reaction and the act, it must also be remembered that many performed acts are themselves but physical exhibitions of memory. Both depend upon the brain or nerve pattern, and we may truthfully state that from the simplest act to the most complex thought our facility depends upon our ability to remember. It depends upon our ability to dip down into our minds and there find, more or less consciously, a brain pattern which shall be useful in the solution of the problem before us. Whether this problem be a whistling for the dog, or the forming of a judgment on internationalism, we require for its solution a power of recalling appropriate brain patterns.

A good memory, then, consists essentially in the possession of many well-marked brain patterns, with the ability to bring these patterns into action as needed. The process is a double one—a process of recording, and a process of recovery, but the physiological nature of these two steps is similar. The making of the record depends upon (1) the physiological endowment of the brain—the development and impressibility of the neurons, and the length of time an impression tends to remain; (2) the manner of making the impression, its emphasis; and, (3) the number of associations which we can gather around it. The first of these factors is determined by nature and must vary in different individuals. That some will have brain cells which more easily receive and retain impressions than do those of others seems evident; and that some will have brain cells where others have none, seems also evident. Fully developed cells which easily receive and retain all impressions are what constitute a "good natural memory." But this matter of physiological endowment is only one of the factors, and the others, as being more within our control

MEMORY

should interest us the more. It is through these
other factors that we must seek improvement
in memory. The physiological endowment is
a set limitation; it is only by improved *method*
that we can hope for betterment. The situation
is analogous to the training of the victim of infantile paralysis—the destroyed nerves here set
the limits to what can be gained, but, by the
training, the patient may be taught to use what
he has to better advantage.

A good impression implies emphasis, and emphasis is obtained by attention, and attention
may be either a deliberate act of the "will," or
it may be the result of that inclination and
"willingness" which we call interest. Attention, from a physiological standpoint, we may
describe as a flow of nerve force, neurokyme,
into one certain pattern, or group of related
patterns, to the exclusion of all others. Thus,
we "give attention" with our eyes, activating a
visual centre in our brain, refusing to divert the
gaze, and refusing to "pay attention" to the
pictures presenting in the marginal visual
fields. We are reading, for instance, and we
keep our eyes directed to the page; we try to
avoid seeing what is going on around us; and
we "close our ears" to the sound of talking.
The brain areas stimulated are those of vision

79

and of visual word images, the auditory images corresponding to these, and the association areas of thought and reason also related. There is also a leakage of the nerve force into the motor areas associated with the more familiar speech, and with some, to whom reading is an infrequent occupation, the lips will move, as the words are silently articulated. Assisting these perception and association areas are the motor areas which hold and secure our best, most appropriate, and most comfortable body positions; so that we may see well and not be distracted by sensations of fatigue nor of unnecessary effort. This motor reinforcement of our perception areas is especially evident when we are listening with attention to a speaker. We are intent upon his words, we directly face him that the sound may enter both ears equally, or we "give him our good ear," if we have but one; we want to see him that we may gain all possible visual aid to our hearing and understanding—that aid which comes from reading the unspoken language of gesture and facial expression. We gaze at him, and often slightly bend forward, both to get nearer and, also, because this position is an instinctive expression of interest, and of a readiness to act. We sit very still; we may even hold the breath. When we can not see the speaker, and wish very much to hear him, we sometimes close our eyes, thus cutting off the visual impressions which have now become irrelevant to the matter in hand. The whole process is one of activating just such, and only such, brain patterns as are associated, pertinent, and useful.

Idle tapping of the fingers, or the making of other useless movements, roving eyes, and interest in extraneous sounds, all these are, of course, evidence of lack of attention. Says Schopenhauer: "I feel respect for the man who when he is waiting or sitting unoccupied refrains from rattling anything, or beating time—the probability is that he is thinking of something." Attention requires energy and as we have just so much energy available, it must be conserved, not dissipated. Hippomenes, Atalanta, and the golden apples is a fable which applies.

The concentration of seeing and hearing, and the limitation of movement, will naturally go far in bringing about a concentration of thought. The idle thoughts which divert us during study are largely those which have been touched into being by the impressions, or stimuli, brought to us by our wandering sight and hearing. The filling of a boy's study room with

81

souvenirs of his camping trips and of his athletic strivings, is thus adding psychologically to his difficulties. Exclude these pleasant stimuli and foreign thoughts will not so often intrude.

Where there is interest in the subject before us attention is easily given, but where interest is lacking attention is attained to with difficulty. A boy is trying to study—he is not interested; he does not care whether the Ukraine is a country or a musical instrument, it rather sounds to him like the latter, and he does not care whether the Volga flows into the Caspian Sea or the British Channel—an automobile passes, he pricks up his ears, it sounds like a Ford. He wishes that he had a Ford—then he remembers the way Douglas, in the moving pictures yesterday, skipped down the mountain cañon in that machine of his. He would like to do that, especially if a certain girl he could (but won't) mention was looking on—the Volga flows south, and southwesterly—no, southeasterly, into the Caspian Sea—what actress is it whose name sounds like Volga? Oh yes, now he remembers, he saw her in New York—and so on to the end of the study period. How different when the interest is engaged! This same boy who can not possibly remember the height of Mount

Everest will tell you the batting averages of all the leading players in both of the Leagues.

When one is not naturally interested, an earnest effort should be made to concentrate— an earnest, persistent, continued and repeated effort—but one should, also, try to *discover* interests, even where these do not at first seem possible. Interest is largely a matter of getting a thing into some sort of relation to one's self. Suppose a boy is keen about military affairs, all European geography and history can be made to appeal. Suppose he is interested in aviation, or in automobiles, the study of physics may become a pleasure. The successful teacher will discover these interests, these true points of contact with the boy's life and ambitions, and will handle the school studies so as to develop them; but the relations must be actually pointed out, or the average boy will miss them altogether. Boys have cubby-hole minds, each subject is placed religiously by itself; school and his own natural interests are most certainly invariably separated. He can not well conceive of any real interest getting over into the school compartment. He repells the very idea. He may "in private life" be deeply interested in gas engines, and yet find physics a bore—physics belongs to school, it *must* be a bore, the logic is conclusive!

The interest of self-advantage, the rewards of success in examinations and of knowledge stored for use in the future, makes but a poor incentive to study. A boy is concerned only with the present advantages, not with the future, and this thing he has heard, anyway, until he is heartily tired of its sound. It is a too frequent resort of the lazy teacher, and is practically useless.

Finally, however, be it noted, there is an interest, a real one, which comes with knowledge. If we can but hold to a task until we really know something of it, the rest will be easy. The trouble with a boy is that he thinks he knows it all before he has attained to the first little beginning.

We have apparently digressed from the matter of memory, but all this has to do with the formation of that first requisite of the process, the brain impression. Interest and attention must always remain the principal factors in the making of this impression. Concentration and interest applying directly to the pattern being registered, together with a reinforcement by associations, gives us our best mental records. The associated interests entangle, as it were, the otherwise uninteresting fact, making it a part of an interesting system, or complex, and thus hold it in mind.

Where emphasis can not be obtained by interest, either direct or indirect, attention may be aided, and emphasis secured, by a sort of pictorial representation of the matter in hand. But before illustrating this idea, let me refer briefly to the second part of the memory process, the act of remembering.

If we assume a recorded brain pattern, *remembering* consists in directing to this pattern a nerve force of sufficient strength to again waken it into activity. Close attention may again be necessary. We are now concerned with that which is within, so we close our eyes, "shut our ears," and sit very still, as we grope around in our minds—to do what? Either to find directly the pattern sought, or to get hold of something which will lead us to it. Practically it is almost invariably by the second method, by associations, that we do finally arrive at the desired pattern, and the more associations there are, the greater the number of connecting threads, the more likely we are in our gropings to find what we want. The evil of *cramming* lies in this, that, while by concentrated study brain impressions can be made, these impressions, not having been oriented and associated with other brain patterns, remain isolated, and soon sink beyond the possibility of recovery. *Forgetting*, then, consists essentially in not having a sufficient number of associations by which a fact may be recalled. *Remembering wrongly* is quite another matter. Here, associations are made, but they are wrong ones—they are the products largely of an unconscious mental action which has been determined by some form of prejudice.

Let us apply some of these concepts of the memory function. I have mentioned the picturing of a fact which we desire to remember—this, and the formation of appropriate associations, are the simple and practical aids. One man ties a knot in his handkerchief to help him remember to call up Smith on reaching his office. Another has a string tied to his finger by his wife that he may not forget to bring home the candy. These are artificial associations deliberately formed. The ancient Peruvians kept all manner of elaborate records by means of knots (quipus) tied in cords of divers colours. Pictorial representation and association are, in one way or another, at the root of all "memory systems," these being really only more or less intelligent conscious exaggerations of the normal brain processes.

Picture what you want to remember; make a vivid picture; make it large, caricature it if necessary. To take a few very simple examples —you always forget whether *until* has two *l*'s or one. Picture the word printed large on a sheet of paper, with two *l*'s, and then picture a heavy black line drawn through the last one. You always forget whether *tendency* has two *e*'s, or an *e* and an *a*. Picture the word on paper, with a very large *E* in the second place. You want to remember the date of the union of Scotland with England—think of the boundary of the two countries, and then picture a great sign, like a modern advertising sign, with the figures 1 6 0 3 stretching across.

You may also usefully combine your pictured fact with certain simple associations which you know will naturally come to mind at the time the fact will be needed. You have an examination tomorrow and you want to remember the date of the fall of the Bastile—picture the blackboard which you will then sit facing, and picture upon it, in large figures, the date, 1789. When you face that blackboard on the morrow the date will be there, in a mental association with it. You are to stop on your way home, to get a can of tomatoes—picture to yourself a mammoth can of tomatoes on the pavement in front of the grocery. You will find that you can not pass the spot without the picture recurring to you. Associate a certain mail-box, one you are to pass, with the letter now in your pocket, and you will mail the letter when you come to the box. Many a mail carrier has been converted into a postman by this simple plan.

These suggestions may sound trivial and artificial, but they are neither, they are but adaptations of nature's own way. You go into the next room to get something, and you forget what you went for, so you come back to where you were sitting when you formed the wish; you there pick up some unconscious thread of association, and now you remember. Why not then make deliberate, conscious associations round the fact to be remembered, associations such as shall be likely to come to mind when needed? The picture, too, is a nature method; we doubtless do naturally form these pictures within our minds—why not then do so deliberately? You are to learn Gray's "Elegy." Picture the scenes as they develop in the poem; picture the tolling bell, picture the herd coming slowly over the lea, picture the ploughman plodding toward his home, picture the gathering twilight—make the poem real, not a mere succession of words; you will remember it the better, and it will have acquired new values.

In remembering a long list of items, associate them in pairs. You are to remember certain things, *A, B, C, D,* and *E*—things to do, things to say, points of an address, things to get. Remember *A* and *B* in relation to each other, making a picture of them together; then, *B* and *C,* in relation to each other in another picture, distinct from the last; then *C* and *D,* in like manner; and then *D* and *E;* each time dropping the previous combination, and not bothering with the next until you come to it. Look now around the room and associate a series of objects in this way. You will find that in a few moments you can memorize, say, twenty objects, which series you can repeat forward or backward without any difficulty.

Another application of this same "chain association" is to link up our items to be remembered with the units of some other series already known and easily recalled. For instance, you know well the arrangement of your room—think of the things in it in a certain order. Starting at the door, we will say we have—a chair, a table, the bed, an electric light, the bureau, a shelf of books, and so on. You have a number of errands to be remembered. Associate these errands with the objects in your room, in the order named. You are to go down town and want to buy a hat, an umbrella, a pad of writing paper, and some pencils; and you want to order a taxi for the evening, and you want to get tickets for the theatre. Associate the hat with the chair; make a mental picture of the hat on the chair. The umbrella you picture on the table; the pad of paper, on the bed; the pencils you hang from the electric light. The taxi you represent in miniature on your bureau, and the tickets you see sticking out from your books on the shelf. When you go to town recall the chair, the table, the bed, etc., to mind—the associations you have made with these will come too, you can not escape them. One of the "systems" of memory now being largely advertised is founded on this principle, which it has developed most skilfully.

In most of what has been said I have assumed the usual visual type of memory. Some of us, however, remember better by hearing than by seeing, and will, therefore, have to adapt the foregoing suggestions; using, as it were, auditory pictures, or auditory and visual combined. I speak of types—as a matter of fact where the visual memory is bad the auditory is generally bad also, but some do show a preference, and it is upon this preference that the idea of "types" has been based. Rhymes are useful aids to these "auditory memories," as they are, indeed, to all—for how otherwise could we remember the number of days in the month?

Just a word as to *partial memories,* they present some interesting features. A recorded pattern may receive a slight stimulation, and yet not be excited to full activity. The effect to us is that of a near-remembering, a sensation perfectly true to the physiological fact. We may be seeking a name—it is, we say, on the tip of the tongue. Here the desired brain pattern has been partially stimulated, but not sufficiently so to bring it into full consciousness. Had it not been stimulated at all we would have had no such sense of impending knowledge; while had it been fully stimulated the knowledge would have been complete. We enter a room for the first time, and suddenly there comes to us a sense of knowing the room, of having been there before. Here is a partially stimulated memory, for what has happened is that something in the room has suggested some other room we have known. The suggestion is, however, not vivid enough to fully recall that room to our minds; it only partially so recalls it, and we get as the result nothing but a vague sense of familiarity. If the likeness and association and resulting memory are vividly real, then we say at once, "Oh, this looks like So-and-so's room!" This phenomenon is not an evidence of a wandering of our spirit, nor of a former incarnation.

Physiologically and psychologically, memory is a comparatively simple process—it is because of its practical importance that I have given it so much space. Important in itself, it is, also, the foundation of most of our other mental processes. Without it, for example, *imagination* would be impossible. We can not imagine that which we do not know. We can not imagine a new colour, nor a new sound, nor a new anything; we can only rearrange such patterns as we already possess, and thus make new combinations out of our memory store. The highest mental process of all, *thought* itself, is dependent upon the memories available.

CHAPTER VII

KNOWLEDGE AND INTELLIGENCE

KNOWLEDGE, if we assume intelligence, depends upon opportunity. It is in the nature of an accomplishment. Intelligence is a matter of capacity, and depends upon the inheritance of brain cells, upon their development, and especially upon their development in the pathways of association. In these days of increasing demands upon the individual in the competition of life, it has come to be recognized that the intelligence is the factor of moment. Knowledge is secondary and, if lacking, may be easily provided. The old knowledge tests of society and the schools are now felt to be inadequate. What we want to know is, not how many facts an individual has managed to accumulate, but his attitude toward these facts, and his ability to make them useful. We wish to know his power and quickness in making mental adjustments, his keenness of perception—in short, his understanding.

So has been born the Intelligence Test—the Binet Test—a test not of knowledge, but of mental adaptability, and of mental efficiency. Knowledge and experience are eliminated so far as is possible. It has not been a simple problem, and the tests as we have them today are far from perfect, but it is an important move, and in the right direction. The ideal is to obtain a series of standards by which the child or the adult may be accurately graded, as normal, subnormal, or superior. If not normal, the degree of abnormality should be possible of determination and record. So far, the tests are of little value other than in childhood, and it may easily be that this limitation will remain. With adults the old mental tests and the new intelligence tests, having made all due allowance for conditions, will be found to yield fairly parallel results, and the importance of the intelligence test here seems to rest simply in its broader application and in its freedom from dependence upon the particular kind of knowledge each individual may happen to possess. Opportunity for acquiring knowledge is now so universal that failure to avail one's self of it is, in itself, evidence of deficient intelligence. With the child the problem is different, and here the intelligence test has proved of real value.

By the examination of many thousands of children, it has been determined what may be reasonably expected from a child of any given age. The child that departs considerably from this average expectation is regarded as abnormal—a child of fifteen, for instance, who can attain only to the expected average for a child of eleven is counted defective. This classification, of course, can not be a hard and fast one, it being obvious that allowances must be made for differences in rate of development, as well as for the influence of various extraneous factors. Children over nine years of age are, therefore, not counted defective unless they rank in intelligence at least three years behind their chronological age; while children under nine are so considered when but two years behind. It has been found convenient to classify and name those defectives with an intelligence age below two, as *idiots;* those with an intelligence of between three and seven, as *imbeciles;* and those who range from eight to twelve, as *morons.* But note that this classification is for convenience only; there are no actual dividing lines. From the drivelling idiot to the master mind one passes by insensible gradations.

These defectives, it will be remembered, are all cases of too early cessation of growth in the association areas of the brain. Possibly from some severe illness in infancy, but generally from some primary lack in the vital urge, the impulse toward continued development within the brain is lost, sometimes suddenly, but in others, and more frequently, after a slowing down stage which may cover several years. Thus a child may be normal to five years of age, and then the development may begin to lag, until at eight he may have attained to a mental growth of but six. He has spent three years in advancing one—and he may go no further, he may remain at six, and be classed henceforth as a high-grade imbecile. I have spoken of primary lack of the vital urge, and of severe illness in infancy. In the case of the latter, one generally thinks of inflammatory disease of the brain itself, but it should be noted that there are many cases of mental retardation which are neither congenital nor due to these inflammatory processes. Mental development may be seriously retarded by disease of any organ, and is often notably so by disease of the ductless glands. There is here a glimmer of hope for the mentally defective, and doubtless, as our knowledge advances, more and more of these cases will be reclaimed to the normal life.

Space can not be spared here for the intelligence tests themselves, but a caution may be uttered as regards their interpretation. In studying the results of any such test all possible influencing factors must be considered. Heredity and all physical and economic conditions must be taken into account. Poor food, insufficient food, unhappy home conditions, chronic or frequent illness, catarrh, adenoids, errors of vision, etc., all necessarily lower the apparent intelligence. On the other hand *noblesse oblige,* and so does good food, warm clothing, a happy comfortable home, and good health. While a child with physical and home difficulties will probably measure below his true level, a child happily situated should be expected to measure "high."

We are dealing here with a matter of great social importance. Society presents all grades of intelligence. Some are remarkable in their quick understanding and in their ready adjustment to the most highly complex problems; others do well in ordinary affairs, but fail when faced by the unusual. Others, again, are efficient only in the simplest of situations; while some, alas! are confused and non-plussed even by these. Dr. Goddard tells of a girl who had learned to make a bed alone, but who was thrown into confusion by the proffer of help.

The superior intelligences are unfortunately few, and the mass of the population measures disappointingly low. It would seem as though social revolution had outstripped the slow evolution of the brain, leaving us behind, as it were, and no longer able to measure up to what our complex modern life demands. Only the exceptional man can be said to be fully efficient today; the rest of us must be satisfied with something less than full efficiency. Charles Francis Adams was very near the truth when he said that "a man ought to be satisfied if he can get through life without making a conspicuous ass of himself."

It has been frequently stated in this book, that social institutions are normally the product of the individual need, that they are outgrowths from man's necessities. This being true, one would reasonably expect that society could never confront man with problems beyond his capacity. Society, the creature, should not be beyond the understanding and control of the average man, its creator. This would indeed be the case had society evolved *pari passu* with man, but there have entered disturbing factors, factors not evolutionary, but revolutionary. I refer to invention and discovery. What one exceptional man may do, may, in its far-reaching social influence, derange the whole of the social growth, and give it, by increased impetus, or side-thrust, a movement different from or far beyond that possible by evolution alone. The fifteenth century's printing, the sixteenth century's voyages of discovery, and the nineteenth century's steam and electricity have been the most serious of these disturbing influences, and have resulted in completely breaking the normal parallel between man and society. They are the "faults," to use a geological term, which have broken the continuity of the social strata. The greatest of these is steam.

One hundred and fifty years ago, an intelligence test based upon the then required efficiency would have graded the populace much higher than does the corresponding test today. Man has gone on his slow evolutionary way, and the man of today is probably a little more intelligent than was the man of yesterday; but society, too, has gone on, and not by any slow biological creeping, but by a series of leaps and bounds. Man's movement is almost imperceptible; that of society is saltatory. Rapid inter-communication has speeded up life to a degree beyond measurement, and man has been left in the lurch. No wonder the world is in a state of unrest! Man is being dragged, like a child by its thoughtless hurrying mother—its arm is fairly out at the socket. Only in this case it is society, the child, that is doing the dragging, and its elderly parent is the one that is breathlessly trying to keep up.

What do we find in the working world? Some occupations, the skilled trades, for instance, require much training, and but little intelligence; while others, such as the executive positions, require little training, and much intelligence. Here lies the explanation of the large salaries paid to executives, and so resented by labour. Executive intelligence is rare, the ability to labour is common. It is merely a question of supply and demand. Here too lies the failure of government management where the executive, important, and difficult positions are filled by political favour; and here lies the explanation of the breakdown when labour itself assumes control. Witness the early efforts at Bolshevist control of industry in Russia, and the quick destruction resulting. It is perfectly proper to wish that labour might have a hand in the conduct of affairs, but the fact is, as it seems to a psychologist, the hands of a factory would be about as badly off without an intelligent control, as would be the hands of the body without their head employer.*

* For an exposition of one phase of the modern labour-capital problem, the division of reward, see Æsop: *The Belly and the Members.*

100

KNOWLEDGE AND INTELLIGENCE

I may seem to be intruding personal views in social economy, but I believe in psychology, and feel that the political economists, who are at least partially responsible for the present world mess, can hardly be counted on to get us out again by any further experimenting. It seems to me that there must be a complete re-orientation of thought, and that our problems must be approached fundamentally and not through political formulas.

In government, as in industry, leadership looks easy—government looks easy. Intelligence does not sweat at its labour, or it does so only in private, and it is therefore unappreciated by the masses. In our democracy, training is conceded to be necessary for an engineer or a fireman, but executive and legislative positions are supposed to be open and possible for all. Democracy will never become what it ought to become, until this error of attitude is corrected. This is no undemocratic class distinction I am making, at least none in the sense of favouring any particular caste; intelligence is to be found in all walks of life, and is by no means especially prominent with the rich. *It is not that Cleon is unfit to rule because he is a worker in leather—it is simply that his fitness must be otherwise determined.*

Since so few of us are intelligent enough to be efficient in many lines, it has become important to discover those in which we can do our best work. To meet this necessity there has come into being a new, practical, Occupational Psychology, an attempt, by various tests, to determine a man's most promising field of endeavour. There is a real tragedy in being in the wrong position. Many a man goes through life on a very humble plane, who might have been distinguished had he had but the fortune to get properly placed in the beginning. Youth does not often have an intelligently directed ambition, and, even when youth has, mistakes are still inevitable, for conditions outside of ourselves generally determine the road we must travel. Accidents largely determine both the ambition and the possibility in starting a career; it is a fortunate man who both knows what he wants and is able to go after it. The new occupational psychology aims to reduce the number of errors by advising whenever a choice seems possible.

CHAPTER VIII

THOUGHT AND JUDGMENT

IT is a common saying that but few people think. Well, that depends—from the standpoint of the position taken in this book, thought is a common possession of all men, and is even shared by them with other of the higher animals. The possession of a brain implies certain mental processes, and these, in turn, imply thought. All will concede, for example, that animals have memory; but thought, I shall claim, is a mere elaboration of memory; it is memory glorified by rich associations, as I believe I can show. Physiologically, thought may be conceived of as a flowing of the nerve force into available brain patterns; and its possibility therefore depends upon the existence of these patterns. The value of thought is, of course, another matter. When we come to consider values then we have to take into account the degree of development and also the matter of thought symbols. Thought, to be perfected, must find an expression, and language is one of its main elements.

Man's thought is thus conceived as differing from that of less endowed animals in quality rather than in kind; it is a difference in the number of available brain patterns, accentuated by a difference in language. A dog speaks with his bark, his growl, his whine, and, also, with his ears, the hair of his neck, his body attitude, and, last but not least, with his tail. He can tell of anger and fear, of elation and abasement, of hunger, and of pleasure and pain—he can even invite his master to go out for a walk. A bird sings love melodies to his mate, and woos by sweet song and by enticing display of his plumage. All this is language, and very sincere in its character, but it is limited in scope. A dog's tail is more to be trusted than is the word of many a man, but he can not lay before us the reasons for his opinion. Animal language, as a rule, is expressive of general ideas only, and is distinctly emotional; the finer intellectual elaborations can not be made. With man it is different; he has acquired a great variety of symbols expressive of many things, and these he uses to talk with, and these he uses to think with. "Thoughts are a kind of mental smoke and require words to illuminate them." *

I have said that a dog tells of his emotions—

* Tom Paine.

a man, too, may use dog language to tell of his. The gesture, the exclamation, the facial expression often reveal thoughts which words may be used but to conceal. Elaborate intellectual processes, however, requiring the use of word symbols and a highly developed brain, have become possible to man, and to man only. Unfortunately, man has not always treated language with the respect it deserves. Small mentalities degrade it; and carelessness does the same, with a resulting degradation of mentality. When a person has but two or three adjectives, such as *splendid, grand, terrible,* and *rotten;* when one *loves* or *hates* everything one comes into contact with; these words cease to be parts of speech, they become but emotional expressions marking approval or disapproval. When a girl describes everything from a necktie or a puppy, to the' League of Nations, as *grand,* she is but metaphorically wagging her tail. This is a reversal of the evolutionary uplift; it is an exhibition of catabolism, of the breaking down of the language accomplishment, and can but have its limiting effect on thought.

Let us follow some of the thought processes and get an idea of what they consist. A man is undressing; he unbuttons his waistcoat, and takes off his watch, and begins to wind it. These actions are all automatic, there is no stimulation of consciousness—but suddenly there is a grating sound, and he can turn the stem no further. The nerve pathway, A, B, C, D, is broken, we will say at C. The habitual pattern is interrupted, and consciousness is at once stimulated. Instead of flowing on automatically and unconsciously to D, the nerve force is blocked and must flow elsewhere. It goes, we will say, to X, where there is a vague picture of the works and their workings. It is recognized that something is wrong—and the current flows to Y, which is a memory of having dropped the watch. From Y, it goes back to X, and then to M, who is a jeweller and watchmaker to whom the watch must be taken in the morning.

So far, it is evident, we are dealing with a process of associative memory, and yet we are also at the beginning of thought. The picking up of consciousness at C, where our automatic pattern was interrupted, and the running of the nerve force here and there into associated areas, is a thinking process comparable with reverie, though with a purposive direction which is lacking in this latter.

If we now introduce the idea of *choice*, we

come to a higher plane. Suppose, in our
example, we reach not M alone, but L, M, and
N, all watchmakers. Before the mental act can
now be completed, a choice must be made. Now
begins a comparison and weighing; the nerve
force flows backward and forward, each time
developing new details of the patterns presented. L is good, but high priced; M is too
far away. N is handy, but has an unpleasant
manner. Well, M is far away, but you can take
a car to the door. As regards N, however, why
should we care about the manner of the man if
he does his work well? And so on, until the
choice is made. This we may call *deliberative
thought*, but it is still memory, we are but looking over our past experiences to find one which
will fit the present case and thus enable us to
act. The process is the same whether the problem be simple or complex, and whether the end
be a mere choice or an elaborate judgment.
The nerve force flows from one pattern to another; meeting an obstruction it flows back, or
is diverted and seeks new pathways; but it
tends always to flow on, here and there, until it
finds that pattern which answers the problem.

If the right pattern be not found, most of us
must then abandon the problem. A highly
developed brain, however, will not yet concede

failure, and will now proceed to another of its resources. Where no suitable pattern can be found already existing, there remains, for some, the further possibility of constructing a new pattern entirely—taking a part of one old one here, and a part of another there, until, finally, from many such parts a new design is made, one which will truly satisfy the requirements. This is *constructive* or *original thought*. It is, we may say, guided memory, plus imagination, plus many brain patterns.

The nerve force flows until it finds the *right pattern*. What is a right pattern? We may answer, I believe, that it is one which is not contradicted by any other. What is true for us, in an intellectual way, is that which finds within us no contradicting brain pattern—that which arouses no sense of conflict, that which finds no opposition; that which is free, therefore, to work unhampered by any contrary tendency. A child looks out of the window, and sees snow for the first time—he exclaims, "Oh, look at the sugar!" Later he gets some new patterns pertaining to snow, and learns that it is cold, and not sweet; but when the original judgment was uttered these contradictory experiences did not exist, and the first judgment was, therefore, both satisfactory and "true." All the facts possible must be obtained before forming a judgment; a pattern may be true in a dozen respects, and yet these may all be negatived by a single addition. I describe a person I have just met—red face, no moustache, rather small features, a heavy drinker—and you form a picture. I add that the person is a baby, and your picture is shattered. Comment on this obvious essential in the making of judgments may seem unnecessary, but I once read of an identification by the police, where the prisoner had so many points of resemblance to the man wanted, that the single fact that his eyes were of a different colour was not permitted to acquit him.

The value of a judgment, then, will depend upon the number of patterns one has available, but it will also depend upon the use one makes of these patterns. Let us assume two men with exactly the same patterns. Their thoughts may differ greatly in value, and will so differ, according to their powers of appreciating and using their pattern material. One will fail to see conflicting elements, which the other will see at once; or will see them in unessential differences which the other will recognize as unessential. Again, one may fail to find any pattern which suits the case, but the other will see that a certain complex contains, in its hidden parts,

109

just what is needed. One is a superficial thinker; the other, a keen thinker—they have the same patterns, but they use them with very different effect. It is a matter here of the development of the association areas, and this, we may confidently state, lies at the root of all variation in thought values. Other, non-intellectual, causes for variation in the value of judgments will be spoken of later. Strictly speaking, of course, the pathways through the association areas are included in the complete brain pattern, but in the assumption made here, that the two men possessed the same patterns, we have limited the meaning of the latter to the registered experiences. We have assumed that they have had the same experiences and the same education—in other words, that they have that kind of likeness which is appreciable to others.

There is a sort of physiological satisfaction whenever a "true" answer is obtained to a problem. The successful completion of a nerve circuit produces a pleasing feeling just as do all successfully carried out physiological acts. It is furthermore important to note that the satisfaction is the same whether the thought has involved many patterns or few, and that, in fact, it may be the more complete in the latter case. , The right pattern, we found, was one which met with no contradiction from other patterns—but, the fewer the patterns the less likelihood of such contradiction. If one has but few patterns, and these not closely connected, they are not likely to clash, and the decision made is a pure one, and consequently eminently satisfying. Where, on the other hand, the patterns are many, a decision may easily carry with it a sense that some of them were open to suspicion, that they contained elements which, it may be, deserved closer attention than had been given. We think we are right, but maybe we are wrong. Our decision becomes a qualified decision and lacks, therefore, that complete satisfaction which we accord to "truth."

The less experience, then, we have had of a subject, the easier it is to arrive at a judgment concerning it, and the greater our satisfaction in that judgment. The three stages of intellectual development may be designated as, *confidence, inquiry,* and *doubt,* and the last, the highest, the doubtful stage, will make decisions far more justly than will the first, the stage of cocksureness. The difficulty in this highest stage is in obtaining a sufficient confidence to insure action—and action of some kind is the real end of thought. Herein lies the essential difference between youth and age. Youth is foolish, but acts; and though generally wrong does sometimes stumble on truth. Age is wise, but doubts; and to it action seems hardly worth while. Youth is radical and ignorant, but does things; age is conservative and experienced, but impotent. Montaigne was right when he said that, "Maturity hath her defects, as well as greenenesse, and worse;"

"First we get Power, but Power absurdly placed
In Folly's keeping, who resigns her charge
To Wisdom when all Power grows nothing worth:"*

From childhood up we are, for the reasons I have given, all satisfied with our judgments, and they are, moreover, very precious to us. To quote Montaigne again: "We easily grant in others the advantage of courage, of bodily strength, of experience, and of beauty, but we yield the advantage of judgment to nobody." Nature has been generous in her gift of understanding, for there is no one but is contented with the share she has allotted him. "The way of a fool is right in his own eyes." So true is this, that a wise man may learn from a fool, but a fool from a wise man, never.

* Browning.

112

THOUGHT AND JUDGMENT

It is the *conceit* of the mentally defective that excites criticism and impatience in those before whom they parade their shallow judgments. One does not criticize a lame man, but one would if the lame man were vain of his physical perfection. It is the vanity we criticize in a fool, not his foolishness—and yet, rightly looked at, his vanity is but a part of his foolishness.

A child will bow to authority and still feel that he is right in his own view of the case. He knows he can do it; he knows he won't break it; he knows he won't hurt himself; he knows it won't make him sick. His facts may be few —he will grant that—but his opinion, he feels, is as good as any one's. When we do accept the judgment of others it is either because the problem does not touch us personally, does not interest us, or, because it is one so far removed from our experience that we do not attempt a judgment for ourselves. The attitude of the public toward scientific affairs is an example in point; as is, also, the old-time attitude toward theology. When inquiry begins, however, and, with it, reasoning, then we make our own judgments and henceforth scrutinize those of others most critically. Note the modern attitude toward the church, as compared with the old.

PSYCHOLOGY OF THOUGHT AND FEELING

Note the birth of the so numerous sects when the lid of priestly authority was lifted by Luther.*

Between absolute acceptance of another's judgment, and absolute rejection of the same, lies half-hearted acceptance. Here the judgment presented to us is accepted, but at the same time there is partially aroused, somewhere in our subconscious collection of brain patterns, one which is antagonistic. If this antagonistic pattern had risen to full consciousness, we would have rejected the judgment, but being only partially stimulated the full antagonism is not perceived—we accept the judgment accordingly, but with an uncomfortable sense of dissatisfaction, with a feeling that something is wrong. In wilful insincere rejection, on the other hand, we recognize the truth intellectually, but shut our eyes to it, and make an emotional denial—the intellectual truth being contrary to some deep-seated prejudice.

If we are all so satisfied with our own understanding, how then are we to attain to wisdom? How are we to know wisdom when we see it?

* The multiplication of new creeds following the Reformation was not, however, due solely to the freedom of discussion. Its deeper foundation lay in the release of the diverging desires and dispositions of men, and in the subsequent formation of groups of the like-minded. That it required many groups, many churches, to provide for all, was to be expected.

THOUGHT AND JUDGMENT

Ulysses exclaims to Athenae, "To know thee truly through all thy changes is given only to those whom thou hast been pleased to grace." Or, as Schopenhauer puts it, "Intellect is invisible to the man who has none." As a matter of fact there is just one hope for us, and that lies in the recognition of our limitations. We must be free to confess that our judgment may be wrong, no matter how right it may seem to us. And *we must learn to judge judgments;* we must learn to look for, recognize, and value the factors involved. Coleridge gives good advice when he says: "Until you are sure of a writer's ignorance presume yourself ignorant of his understanding." Confucius long ago taught that, "to know what we know, and to know what we do not know—this is wisdom." Proverbs has it, "The way of a fool is right in his own eyes, but he that is wise hearkeneth unto counsel." What Confucius and Solomon have said of wisdom applies equally to knowledge, for the mind, however small it may be, completely fills its own field. The ignorant mind is a complete mind so far as it goes, and it carries that same satisfaction which accompanies all completeness. To realize truly how little one knows, and to be dissatisfied with this lack, is the beginning both of knowledge and of wisdom—it signifies much. The savage who knows naught but his own primitive life is well pleased therewith, and, even when brought into contact with the comforts of civilization, experiences no envy—not even wonder; these things are beyond his understanding and interest. It is so with the ignorant mind. When man comes to realize and lament his deficiency, however, then striving begins, and from now on he is neither primitive nor ignorant.

If we can but know our limitations, then, we are already a long way on the road to wisdom. Let us represent wisdom by a fraction—we surely can not aspire to more; unity here would be omniscience. If we write our ability for the numerator, and make the denominator our pretension, it is evident that the value of the fraction can be raised, either by increasing the former, or by decreasing the latter.

But this is not all. The satisfactory working out of any problem requires that we shall approach it with an open mind. We must endeavour to separate the problem from our prejudices! If we start out with an idea which we wish to prove; if we start out, in other words, with the answer; we are pretty sure to find that same answer. Proof of what we wish to believe is easily obtained. What is it we do when we make these prejudiced judgments? We go to our filing-case of experiences and we look it over, and we take from it a fairly large assortment of *what we want*. The other experiences we reject and—Lo! the problem is solved! We have more or less wilfully forced conflicting patterns out of consciousness, and we may ultimately forget them, and come to believe our judgment to be actually true.* This is much as the world has gone to that rich storehouse, the Bible, and has drawn from it whatsoever it has desired—prohibition and wine drinking, celibacy and marriage, polygamy and monogamy, Presbyterianism and Universalism.

I speak of prejudiced judgments as being made by the rejection of conflicting patterns. It is, however, evident that a judgment may be prejudiced in character (that is, unguided by sufficient evidence) and yet, owing to the limitations of the individual, there may really be no conflicting patterns present. Such a judgment is satisfying to its possessor to the highest degree—it is the kind men are willing to die for. Contradict such a judgment and you are met with silent scorn. Contradict, on the other

---

* In a similar way, the force of an epigram lies in the fact that its happy expression temporarily distracts our attention from conflicting patterns, making it, for the moment, as true as it is pleasing.

hand, a judgment where conflicting patterns are present but wilfully ignored, and you are met with anger. Those attempted-to-be-forgotten patterns lying there unused can not be repressed by any intellectual act, they can be reacted against only emotionally. Contrast with these the reaction to criticism where the judgment is purely an intellectual one. Criticism here leads only to argument—men do not die for opinions so coldly conceived.

What are the factors which determine our prejudices, our pre-judgments? They are our innate dispositions and emotions, our temperament, and the influences of group opinions—of *our* group, the customs and attitudes of thought which constitute *our* mores, the mores of *our* family, set, city, state, and nation. Democracy, for instance, is so firmly entrenched with us, that we are hardly capable of discussing it intelligently; it has obtained for us almost a moral value. And yet, to Thomas Carlyle it meant but a form of government in which Jesus and Judas were given an equal vote—a state of affairs he indignantly repudiated. Moral? Yes! Mores—the same word, the same thing! Morals are mores which have become sanctified by long usage; and other mores than ours are—immoral.

We began this chapter with a criticism of the statement that few people think, but if we change that to the assertion that few people make valuable judgments, we shall not be far from the truth. With very many all actions and attitudes are determined by prejudice, without inquiry, and with blindness to the experience of others. These prejudices are like stained-glass windows (Chesterton has suggested the idea) behind which we live and through which we must view the world—very darkly stained they are for some, less so for others. We, each of us, must look through our own windows; we can not get away from them, nor can we see through the windows of others. It would seem that the best we can do is to remember that the windows are there. And yet— all of the stain is not ''burnt in the glass,'' some of it may be cleaned away—education may help. As a matter of fact, education, properly applied, is a wonderful agent. It is education which helps us to control our primitive and subconscious impulses, and it is education, then, which we may bring in to help clean our windows—but it can not do everything, some colour will always remain. Will it be objected that some educated men are noted for prejudice? Well, I make no claim of patent universal efficiency in the agent I advertise. Some colours *are* burnt in the glass, and these permanent colours may be very dark ones. What is truly of serious importance here is, that narrowness of vision, strong prejudices, and dogmatism, especially if accompanied by facility in the expression of idealistic platitudes, makes a whole which seems to the foolish most admirable. A man so unfortunately endowed may easily become a leader, and his limitation of judgment a social menace.

.   .   .   .

In this writing I have endeavoured to avoid speculation, and yet in this presentation of thought and judgment I fear that I have been getting close to debatable ground. That thought should be limited by that which is already in the mind; that it is but a directed voluntary memory; and that the problem should be solved only by recalling, remembering, and examining—all this may seem highly disputable. It is, however, the very foundation of the well tried and proven Socratic method, and to educate—"to draw out"—certainly implies that the something to be drawn out must be already within. New patterns we do truly accumulate, but these must become assimilated with patterns already existing or they remain

120

worthless for reasoning purposes. It must further be realized that I have been describing these processes, not offering explanations. An attempt at teleological exposition would indeed lead us into metaphysical regions.

Just a word more. There is a tendency in science to *identify* all mental processes with their physical origins and thus to abandon the older differentiation of mind and matter. This is what is known as monism—materialistic monism. Now materialistic monism is useful as a working hypothesis—I have so used it in this writing—but it would be wrong to regard it as a scientifically established fact. That consciousness has a reality of its own to the degree that it is capable of modifying physical function, must certainly be granted. The brain is an organ and, materialistically, it can not be different from other organs, but we know that organs alter with need, and even atrophy and disappear when the need is no more. Our own bodies contain many of these vestiges. This is no sophistical argument; it is one which can not be escaped from when we think about it rightly, and it should, at least, make us pause before accepting the monist idea. And yet, on the other hand, how very slight a physical change will profoundly alter, or even obliterate, this same mental power. An apoplexy consists in but the leakage of a few drops of blood into the brain substance. Where does the mind go then?—And why? Let us continue to use the hypothesis so long as it remains useful, but let us not go beyond our facts. "Overbeliefs," those which are held without the foundation of fact, are no more true when they come through the gateway of science than when they lack this prestige.

CHAPTER IX

EDUCATION *

It is not proposed to attempt, within the narrow limits of this small book, a treatise on the psychology of education; the subject is too vast. All education belongs to psychology, and all psychology pertains to education. It is in the hope of bettering education that psychology finds its reason for being. But let us consider briefly a few broad educational principles, and thus indicate that general psychological attitude believed to be helpful in securing results.

The purpose of education we will assume to be a preparation for life—a preparation for the labours and discords of life, and a preparation, also, for *life's leisure*. I italicize this last, it is so often forgotten, if, indeed, it be ever remembered—and yet it may easily become the most important of all. What shall a man do with his leisure? How shall he employ his periods of rest? How he does, will demonstrate his character. And what about that enforced rest

---

* While a separate chapter has here been made of certain of the psychological elements which enter into education, Chapters V to X, inclusive, all pertain directly to educational matters.

of old age, that period when man, like Prometheus chained to the rock, has far more leisure than he likes? There are few beings more pathetic than those aged ones to whom time has brought nothing but years; who have never attained to wisdom, and who, having built their whole scheme of life on a frivolous search for entertainment of the senses, find themselves, at last, with their capacity for this kind of entertainment gone. It may be added, too, that the passing of one's leisure is a matter of growing importance. Whether well advised or not, the hours of labour are everywhere being curtailed, and man's leisure period correspondingly increased. May it not be that part at least of the world's present unrest is due to lack of preparation for this new condition?

It is life, then, in *all* of its aspects, for which education must prepare. At once two problems present—what shall we teach; and how shall we teach it? Most educational work along psychological lines has concerned itself with the second problem alone; the first has been discussed mainly along unpsychological lines, and has taken chiefly the form of a futile debate between the classicists and the non-classicists.

Let us examine the first of these problems for a moment; it is quite as psychological as the second. Knowledge in some form has been universally regarded as the essential element of the educational goal—and it is, but not that which is commonly called knowledge. We have already made the distinction between knowledge and intelligence, let us keep that distinction in mind. No mere storing of facts, dates, names, etc., is worth while from the psychological standpoint. This type of information may indeed be useful, but it is a poor goal to aim at, and should be regarded only as an incident of true education. A trained adult can acquire in one year what it takes the child ten years to acquire, in this kind of knowledge. Many a man of affairs has had no schooling, no book training in youth, and yet stands today an educated man and a leader, not only in business, but in society generally. He may be prominent in municipal or national politics, or an expert in pictures, or books—what you please! Such a man we call an able man; he is a king among men—a king, a kön-ning, a man who can. This man has knowledge of a special kind. To put it in terms of the brain, he has acquired a store of ready-to-use, associated brain patterns by the aid of which he confidently copes with the problems of life. He is a man of education.

Mental growth consists in the obtaining of

experience which, stored away, becomes available for the formation of new brain patterns and the elaboration of the old; but, be it noted, to obtain this it is not sufficient to have merely lived through a series of events. The useful experience in life, that which can be built up into the brain pattern, is the experience which has been grasped, explained and understood, and which has been oriented in the mind with other experiences. It is not the obvious wealth and variety of life that makes the well-stored mind. No life can be well conceived which does not ·present daily experiences sufficient to amply store any mind open to their reception. The country boy, the shut-in, the recluse, the hermit, even, may accumulate great wisdom; it is all a matter of observation and reflection. The Bible has been many a wise man's sole library.

No mere memory of facts can alone give the efficiency here referred to, and yet, informing facts have in the past been considered the major part of education. Botany, when I went to school, consisted in the naming of plants; and when one had analysed his plant, identified it, and named it, he was through. If one knew the botanical names of the plants in his neighbourhood, he was a botanist, though he might not have even the most elementary knowledge of plant life itself, or of its manifold mysteries and functions.

No wonder, in the old days, a valedictorian was regarded with little confidence or hope. It was a common enough saying then, that honour men were no good in after life. In those days it was not the possession of intelligence that determined the school success; it was the retentive memory, and a willingness to subordinate thought to mere acquisition. It was docility rather than originality that gathered the palms. That the recent trials of the intelligence tests have revealed a pretty close parallel between their results and those of the school examinations, is in itself a suggestive endorsement of the newer educational methods. Intelligence has evidently at last entered the school; and, if this be so, no parent need now look askance at his valedictorian son. The ideas of educational method have advanced. Facts which once were introduced *a posteriori*, by the application of birchen rods, were next poured in at the ear. This marked an improvement, but not enough; so far as results were concerned it was like pouring from a bucket into a narrow-necked vase. The present stage is more hopeful; we now seek, in our better schools, to obtain entrance through the child's understanding. Facts are still given, but they are given enriched by inspiring explanation and association; and they are worked in by the teacher until they become a part of the child's mentality.

This ideal has not yet, of course, been generally realized; but it is recognized, and that is a beginning. Self-sacrificing teachers are everywhere making a brave effort to reach this high goal, and it is to our shame that they receive so little appreciation or support. In these days of tense living the conservation and development of brain power should be, but is not, the nation's most important conservation program. Nor by brain power do we mean scholarship; rather we mean that functional control which shall lead to a better life—for intellectualism alone may be a menace. "Lilies that fester smell far worse than weeds." A perversion of thought may be worse than a lack.

It is with the child that we are chiefly concerned. Childhood is the plastic period of life, and it is then that the fundamentals of character are laid down once for all.

Here is one phase of the situation—listen to Bergson: "Each of us, glancing back over his history, will find that his child-personality, though indivisible, united in itself divers persons, which could remain blended just because they were in their nascent state: this indecision, so charged with promise, is one of the greatest charms of childhood. But these interwoven personalities become incompatible in course of growth, and, as each of us can live but one life, a choice must perforce be made. We choose in reality without ceasing; without ceasing, also, we abandon many things. The route we pursue in time is strewn with the remains of all that we began to be, of all that we might have been." *

The direct significance of this from an educational standpoint is of course obvious—the child must not be abandoned to idle chance in making its choice; it must have the advantage of guidance. We are all, more or less, "moved by desires, as puppets by strings," but let us at least learn somewhat to control these desires. It is this, I take it, which is the great aim of education in childhood. Tendencies thrive or remain dormant according to the environment. Of the many possibilities with which the infant begins life, those which will develop will be, generally speaking, those which in his experience (environment) he finds useful. The seeds of thousands upon thousands of dispositions are sown,

* Bergson: *Creative Evolution.*

129

but those only flourish which find a favourable soil.

The child is a most difficult human problem, the developing and understanding of which should call forth all the ingenuity and enthusiasm of research. Unfortunately, many have yet to learn that the problem exists. Wilfred Lay * compares teaching with the driving of an automobile. How much one can get out of a machine depends upon how much one knows of the machine. Any one can drive if the machine works well; it is when it begins to "miss," and otherwise "act up," that the ignorant driver becomes helpless. Such a one will then probably blame the machine, and let it go at that; but another, who knows the machine, will be stimulated by the problem presented, and will generally solve it, possibly by some simple adjustment. Again, the mere driver, through failure to recognize ominous signs, and by endeavouring to force the machine when he should not, may bring about irreparable injury—injury which an intelligent handling would have entirely avoided.

Let us drop any specific application in our use of the word *teacher*, and let us understand that what we have to say pertains to the home

* *The Unconscious Mind of the Child.*

as well as to the school. Certainly the parents are solely responsible for that period of life which is the most important of all—the first six years. The child of six is already far advanced in character formation, and if the start has been bad, so much the worse for all concerned—correction will have already become most difficult.

It is in this first period of life that the deepest and most ineffaceable foundations are laid in the unconscious mind, and this fact alone should indicate its importance. *In these first years lies the principal part of all education, the forming and establishing of useful habits.* There is no greater error than that which the world commits when it places knowledge as the goal of childhood, and leaves the acquiring of good habits to the future. "You can not teach an old dog new tricks," expresses a profound psychological truth. The good habits, moral, social, and personal, which may be obtained in childhood, and then only, count more for the happiness and future welfare of the child than does all the knowledge he can gain in a lifetime.

Is this statement too "strong"? I think not, but if I have made it so, it is only because in practice in our schools habit formation has been so sinfully neglected. I do not wish to detract from the value of learning in general, but merely to point out to parents and teachers where it is that their first duty lies.

The formation of habit is a progressive act; it is in line with the child's development. Education in the ordinary sense, on the other hand, is a looking backward. It is an attempt to carry forward-looking youth backward over paths which others have already traversed—and it is this which makes it so difficult. And yet this too is, of course, necessary if in this short life of ours any true progress is to be made. The past must first be made ours if we are to begin our own progress in the present. The school period corresponds, as it were, to the synopsis of preceding chapters often given in a magazine serial—one must read the synopsis to understand that which follows. But habits, judicial, logical, analytical, of concentration, of application, and of control, are what we must really first seek. These form the valuable part of education, the universally applicable part, the part which carries over from school to the life in the world of men. No study has *per se* much value in developing mind, other than through the habit of mind which may be gained in its pursuit. The great contribution of science to the world has been the scientific attitude. The mere facts in the case are very secondary to the manner of approach to these facts. This is not a denying of the specific value of facts—arithmetic is essential to the storekeeper, as are the higher mathematics to the engineer. Latin is helpful in the study of the romance languages, as it is, also, helpful to a correct knowledge of English. Facts all have their specific values, but in comparison with the mind's development, or in aid to it, they remain secondary. What fact or number of facts can equal in value the power to hold one's self to an unpleasant but necessary task? A man who has finished his educational period—if there be any such—has acquired a set of attitudes. What these attitudes are is the measure of his education.

Character depends only partially upon the innate dispositions and the temperament; it depends really, chiefly, upon the reaction between these factors and the environment—and this is where instruction steps in, to aid in determining what this reaction shall be. Whether your child shall grow up disobedient, deceitful, captious, careless, indifferent, vain, selfish, obstinate, whining, tricky, or impudent; or whether he shall be obedient, truthful, considerate, civil, generous, brave, and kind, depends very largely upon you—the parent. Locke says that every man desires for his son virtue, wisdom, breeding, and learning—with a normal child the first three of these are almost solely, and the fourth, largely, within the parent's control.

In most cases, probably, a bad bringing up will be the result of neglect; it will depend upon our sins of omission. But it may also depend upon a wrong attitude, as, for instance, upon the erroneous notions of parents who may be well intentioned but ignorant. Again, some, through "love for the child" and from a wish not to cross it, will permit it to do things which they know to be wrong—things which must be reckoned for, in tears, later on. And, finally, there are those who deliberately foster the child's worst possible traits; who praise and laugh at what are really incipient vices. They coddle and spoil; and exhibitions of temper, of wilfulness, or selfishness, of vanity, are made the subject of the fond parents' boast. Then, to quote Locke again, "When their children are grown up, and their ill habits with them; when they are now too big to be dandled, and the parents can no longer make use of them as playthings, then they complain that the brats are untoward and perverse." *Fond* parents, I have called them—in earlier times *fond* meant *foolish;* how the word came to be applied as it is now, is evident.

EDUCATION

It is this child, born of you and now further moulded, through its entire formative period, by your teachings, who enters school; do not attempt to shift all the responsibility, for the results there obtained, to the school-teacher. What the child learns there is important enough, but it is largely social—emulation, fair play, social adjustment, the rights of others, and the general duties of the larger circle. The beginning of all this should have been ingrafted in the home, but it is further developed in the school playground and in the classroom. All the rest is the parent's part, and the obligation can not be avoided.

From the purely educational standpoint, aside from habit and character formation (though in reality all pertains to these) our first duty is to explain things to the child, to explain what he sees. Or maybe the first duty of all is to teach him to see, to train him in observation, and to train him in inquiry, and thus to store his mind with experiences, the *sine qua non* of intellectual life. Bring him to an appreciation of the things about him, the things of home life. No finer acquisition can be obtained by a child than a realization that the near. things are the things of importance. Too many of us pass through life without this enriching knowledge, and, missing reality altogether, respond only to the allurement of distance. It would seem as though certain schools deliberately cherish the long-distance view. Under the pleasing mask of social idealism they instil an aspiration toward public service; and the home, the unit and very foundation of all social life, is left to become cold and indifferent. The mirage on the horizon alone allures; near things seem prosaic. Again, as the near-thing is the important thing, so is the near-time. "Write it on your heart," says Emerson, "that every day is the best day in the year."

Some of you will say, "Well, my boy certainly does not have to be taught to ask questions!" No, but does he ask these questions for information, or is his questioning but an idle habit? If he does ask for information, are you sure that you know how to answer him? It will take a wise parent to answer questions well! Let me suggest, however, that all questions should not be directly answered. Instruction is often best effected by putting the child, if not too young, in the way of discovering answers for himself. Thus, if you have the knowledge and ability, point out the analogies of nature, and let him discover from the known forces some explanation of the seemingly more mysterious. Introduce him early to the dictionary and encyclopedia, especially to the former. Do not let your boy grow up shying at books, as a colt shies at paper in general; lead him up to them while he is still young, he will find that they are useful, not dangerous.

There is no better road to clear thinking than over the path of a good vocabulary. Words are essential to thought, as we have already seen, and a poor knowledge of words must make for indifferent thinking. But, in your teaching, remember this, too, words are not things, they are but symbols. Words do not *convey* ideas, they merely *arouse* them, and, like experiences, they must be assimilated and appreciated before they become useful. They are valuable only when the thing they symbolize is understood; they can arouse an idea only if the child's mind already contains the making of that idea. Take an example from adult life. When the radical idealist preaches "liberty" to the audience before him, he is interpreted by many as meaning something far different from the beautiful concept of his own intention. With many, the brain patterns responding will be those of license and freedom from restraint. This limitation of language must be ever borne in mind in talking with children; the words used must connect up with the patterns they already possess, and these must be the right patterns. You, yourself, must be intelligent enough to follow the steps of their possibilities of appreciation. All intellectual acquisition is made on the general plan of that interesting story of "The House That Jack Built." It is a serial process involving repeated additions each of which is assimilated and adjusted to that which has gone before.

Certain languages have an advantage over the English as regards their use by children. When *we* wish to name a thing we commonly turn to the Greek or the Latin, and from roots there found, construct a new word—a word which, without a knowledge of these classical roots, has no meaning until explained. With more strictly national languages, such as the German, for instance, a new word will be constructed from old and familiar ones by a process of compounding, and will carry its meaning with it. Thus, in German a genealogist is a *Geschlechtskundige,* a race or family knower; a tragedy is a *Trauerspiel,* a mournful play; the act of making restoration is a *Wiederbringung,* a bringing back. In English we do the same thing in a limited degree; we do speak of a *steam-ship,* and of a *railway,* for instance, but we much more often turn to the classics. The advantage of the English method is great so far as the language is concerned, but it does also complicate instruction—since Greek and Latin have been removed from their former proud place in our school curriculum.

Practically it has been found that there are definite periods in the brain development of the child when certain concepts first become possible. For example, few children have a true conception of morning and afternoon, as real periods of time, before the age of six. The average child does not appreciate the time interval of a week and gives but little time value to the days of the week, before the age of eight; and not until he reaches nine has he any useful concept of months and years. An appreciation of abstracts is rarely possible before twelve —how could it be? Abstracts are but composites of many related attributes, and their conception can only follow experience. If one knows but one kind of goodness any sense of an abstract good must be impossible. Of course a child may *learn* the days of the week at two; he may use any of the above terms, and he may use them glibly; but they will have no experience value for him, and he will not really sense them.

The child's mind, as I have said, must contain the making of an idea before he can grasp it; words alone convey nothing to him. Development is a growth by the *timely* addition of new facts and experiences, which are added to and assimilated to those related facts already possessed. Instead of this judicious feeding, many a child has presented to it great indigestible globs of material which can produce nothing but a mental dyspepsia. So often is this the case that the child ceases to wonder; it chews its educational fodder with pain but without question. The child recites and makes maybe a perfect recitation; but this is often mere chance, the perfect recitation may indicate no better understanding than the one which displays some ridiculous error. One child may say that Ireland is called the Emerald Isle because it is green; and another may say that it is called the Emigrant Isle for the same reason—the difference may be simply a difference in the acuteness of hearing, not of understanding; neither may understand a word of what they are saying—though in this case both might seem to be right. The answers found on examination papers are sometimes illuminating: ''The Puri-

tans found an insane asylum in the wilds of
America." "Pompeii was destroyed by saliva
from the Vatican." "The abdomen contains
the bowels, of which there are five—a, e, i, o,
and u, and sometimes w and y."

It is this attitude of helpless passivity with
the early discovery that it is futile to try to
understand, that is at the root of that feeling,
lifelong with many, that knowledge is an alien,
unpractical thing, a something to be always
kept apart from the affairs of the real world.
The youth turns with relief from the vagaries
of school to the realities of life. The former
are "silly" and generally "over his head," but
the latter are what he has found out and appreciated for himself, and are, therefore, well
within his understanding. Could education proceed hand in hand with the growth of the child's
capacity this false attitude would never be obtained, and educational affairs would take a
place in his life along with the other realities.
Add this difficulty, this too early administration
of educational provender, to that psychological,
physiological, biologic difficulty already spoken
of, that youth is essentially forward-looking
and that education has to do with the past, and
it is no wonder that our schooling falls so far
below our eager expectations.

Remember the age, then, and the capability of the child when you offer instruction! And so, also, in *conduct*—do not expect ten-year-old conduct from a four-year-old child. Moral training, like the physical and the intellectual, must be developed *pari passu* with the growth. Many a so-called bad child is but a backward child unrecognized as such by its parents. With the very young, do not bother about morals at all, confine yourself to the habits, the rest will come along in due time. The morals, it has been said, are the fruits desired, but the habits are the roots and the branches.

One sometimes hears earnest mothers speaking in gentle expostulation with naughty children, holding forth to them the most highly complex abstract sentiments as motives for good behaviour. Results of some kind may be obtained from such talks, but they are not the product of the moral formulas. They are, as a matter of fact, owing to the *sympathetic emotion* aroused within the child, to the bringing into play of this most elemental reaction. A child listening to the saddened voice of the mother, with its unwonted solemnity, is greatly impressed, and becomes itself conscious of an unhappy feeling. This state of affairs becomes to the child something decidedly unpleasant and, therefore, to be avoided in the future. It is not the talk of Heaven, nor the suggestion that we should aspire to grow up to be honourable men, that has impressed the child—had the mother recited the points of the compass in the same tone of voice, with the same unpleasant solemnity, the effect might have been much the same.

Some children have little of the sympathetic emotion—what are we to do with them? Well, we can spank them; that is one way, and a pretty good one, but not often needed. Whatever we do, however, it must be a concrete thing, not an abstract. Shall we reason with them? That depends—the greatest possible discretion must be observed if we are to undertake this method. Reason is more suitably used as the coping stone in the training of morals, than it is for foundation work; though when handled with wisdom it may have its value. You know the child who answers every command, big and little, with, "Why-y-y?" "*Why* do I have to do it?" "*Why* do I have to go to bed?" "*Why* can't I eat it?" "*Why* can't I go?" Well, this child is the product of a too early attempt at reasoning. If the child by nature were amenable to reason, the situation would be different; but remember what has been said of children's judgments—they are always necessarily satisfactory to the child. This being so, the child can not really accept your judgment unless it happens to coincide with his own. He obeys in the end because he must, because he is a child and you are in authority. How often such "reasoning" comes to an end with an exasperated, "Because I say so!" from the parent. Well, then, why didn't you say so in the beginning? To argue every point, to reduce everything to words, makes a captious, tiresome child, and the habit, as it flowers in after life, is not a pretty one! Explain, yes! but do not argue—and it is generally into argument that the process degenerates. I am speaking, of course, of the very young child. A time comes when the child ceases to be a child, and when reason is the proper approach—another fact often forgotten by parents.

This criticism, first of moral reproof and now of reasoning, will be offensive to some, but it is true to the psychology of childhood. The child must be approached in simplicity. All of the potentialities of life are there in that little body, but we must not be deceived into regarding them as actualities, useful *now* to the child.

We have attained so far but to the idea of sympathetic control, which we recognize can be

useful only with sympathetic children. For
others, it is evident, we must evolve some more
concrete method.

Mother Nature has worked out an idea which
may be useful to us, though we can not adopt
it without some change, for she, strange dame,
is more concerned with the race than she is with
the individual—an attitude never met with in
women of smaller family. I refer to the system
of rewards and punishments. As rewards for
good behaviour nature gives us good health and
happiness; as punishments for going contrary
to her directions we get pain, disease, and
death. As has just been said, this plan, especially as regards the punishment, can be
adopted only after change—capital punishments are not what we are after. To hang a
man may really be a good lesson for him, but
it hardly seems worth while. On the other
hand, all of nature's punishments are not capital, and some of them may well be allowed to
stand.

Within certain limits, when not actually hurt-
ful to the child, we should not try to prevent the
natural consequence of a child's act. When a
child, past infancy, tires of its toy and breaks
it, it should henceforth go without. When,
through lazy carelessness, things have been

145

broken or lost, they should not be replaced. When a weekly allowance has been dissipated in wild orgy, on the first day of the week, there should be six days to await a renewal, six days of leanness. These are difficult disciplines for a generous-hearted parent to effect, but the worth of your love for your child must be measured by your success in carrying them out. It is not a high form of love which cares more for the selfish pleasure of giving than it does for the child's future welfare. Viewed rightly these are the safest punishments that can well be conceived of; they are natural, and logical, and instructive. By them may be developed, very early, a true sense of responsibility, a realization of cause and effect, and a general manliness of outlook on life.

Nature sometimes fails us as a model in that her punishment may be too far removed from the offence. She has not found it necessary to consider the finer psychological truths—her children are so many that she can easily spare some, and therefore dares to work crudely. There is no use in telling a child that if he does so and so, by the time he is fifty he will be an ill man. No, for our purpose, the individual's good, *we must get the punishment, or the reward, into close relation with the act calling it*

146

EDUCATION

forth. A close association must be made between the two in the child's mind. A punishment promised for Saturday—a keeping from
play, for instance—for some offence committed
on Monday, does not establish this necessary
relation. Such a postponed punishment has no
deterrent value and, when it comes, it does
harm, for it arouses only a sense of injustice.
These delayed punishments, with their it-hurts-
me-more-than-it-hurts-you banalities, are absolutely psychologically wrong. The punishment,
if it is to be at all, must be close to the
offence.

The same thing, of course, holds for rewards.
The reward, like the punishment, must be immediate, and should generally be spontaneous
—not offered in advance as a bribe. It should
be some spontaneous, pleasant thing which happens as a seeming part of the good thing the
child has just done. A close association should
be made with the preceding act; the reward and
the punishment should seem to fuse with the
act, so that this shall carry, ever after, a pleasant or an unpleasant memory.

As regards the comparative value of arti-
ficially inflicted rewards and punishments,
there is no question but that the former have
the better psychological foundation. In trying

147

to break a bad habit what we are really trying
to do is to break up a certain undesirable brain
pattern; but anything that calls attention to a
pattern tends to emphasize it and make it
stronger. It is as in advertising; within certain
limits even unfavourable comment is often regarded as better than none.

> "The mair they talk, I'm kent the better,
> E'en let them clash."

In something of this same way, punishment will
emphasize a brain pattern; and when the impulse to act comes again, this emphasized pattern is the one which presents itself and determines the act. Of course if the child deliberated
the result would be different, but the child does
not deliberate; he acts on impulse, and realizes
only when it is too late. The persistent manner in which children will repeat certain actions
"in spite of all punishment" is thus partially
explained. It is not in spite of, it is because of
the punishment that the impulsive child so mis-
behaves.

The emphasis obtained by punishment is a
poor preparation for the breaking of a bad
habit. It is most assuredly and particularly
wrong, too, when its purpose is to inspire to

better achievement. To rap a child's fingers will not make it love the piano; to punish for failure in lessons will not inspire a love for books. Nor should lessons be assigned as a punishment—this is fatal! The Puritans used to punish their children by making them read the Bible, and—New England turned Unitarian. Again there are many more ways of doing wrong than there are of doing right, and if punishment be consistent it must also, necessarily, be too frequent. The child, being so constantly in disgrace and finding itself so often in the wrong, becomes sullen, antagonistic, and rebellious. Finally, punishment, in arousing the destructive emotions of fear and anger, is distinctly injurious to health.

Rewards, on the other hand, emphasize the desirable patterns, and this is what we want. As a result, the desirable brain pattern becomes the working brain pattern, and the undesirable one is forgotten. By the reward, furthermore, the child is kept happy; pleasing emotional states are obtained, and these all work for the better health of the child. Digestion is improved; all physiological processes take place under the best possible conditions; and the child's behaviour is correspondingly bettered. So we go round in a happy circle—good behaviour brings reward; reward makes for happiness; happiness makes for good health; and good health makes for good behaviour. Compare this with the vicious circle set up by punishment!

Ruskin says that the greatest efforts of the race are traceable to the love of praise. Praise is one of the most valuable of our rewards. Only brief comment is called for, the value of this powerful appeal to the elemental emotions is felt by all, and a warning only need be sounded. *Do not indulge in unwarranted praise; limit your praise to that which is praiseworthy.* Do not praise, in a normal child, that which is mediocre—above all, do not praise the result of indifferent effort. Where the effort has been great, praise the effort, no matter what the result; but do not praise the result unless it is well worth it. I know of no way of so quickly lowering a child's standards as by unwarranted, unearned praise. It is here we find part at least of the handicap under which the only, and the favourite, child labours. The vanity, the self-sufficiency, and the inefficiency of these unfortunates is largely due to the admiration with which their souls is constantly fed. The tendency of us all is to minimal effort; we are only too ready to stop with that

EDUCATION

which "will do." If what the child has done
unsatisfactorily be praised, why should the
child ever put forth effort to improve?

Under one condition only may unearned
praise be ventured upon, and that is when it has
been previously very infrequent. When this is
the case it is possible that, used judiciously, it
may develop a spirit of emulation and thus lead
the child to better endeavour. The child may be
stimulated to compete with himself—this is true
emulation—he may gain the desire to earn his
own praise. The pleasure of successful competition, healthfully enjoyed, always consists in
the satisfying of one's own ideals. Then, again,
he knows in his heart that he can do better than
he has already done. The praise for his slight
achievement was a novel and pleasant experience, and he determines to surprise people by
showing them what he really can do.

But we nearly all do tend to minimal effort
and are satisfied with that which is good enough.
We start with the typewriter, and we find that
by the hover-and-search-with-one-finger method
we can get our letter written—so we never
learn a better way. Education, however, means
work; the mind can not be developed healthfully in the luxury of praise alone. As well try
to develop your legs by lying in bed and admir-

151

ing them. Nothing can be developed unless resistance has to be overcome. The Montessori method—a pleasant mental massage which has been substituted for exercise—leads nowhere with a *normal* child, but to harm. Here is the handicap of the rich man's son, his coddling through life resulting, in all but the especially praiseworthy few, in a lasting pitiful disability. To work a boy does not mean that you are to make him a drudge; it means, simply, leading him away from the too easy path of indolence; inspiring him not to be satisfied with inferior ideals; praising that which is praiseworthy; and encouraging always to effort. In short, it means living his life with him, and guiding him, as unobtrusively as possible, with the light of your greater experience.*

Indeed, rest is just as important as work, provided that the work has preceded. Studies, like food, must be digested before they can be assimilated; and brain cells tire even more than do those of the muscles. Rest is essential for the mental digestion, as it is also for the cell recuperation. Note, too, that it is in the play time of the child that there comes your very best opportunity for the laying of his character habits. In play the child is really himself, and

* Read Roosevelt's *Letters to his Children.*

it is in his play that he can be best studied and helped.

Emerson remarks that no one can do anything well who does not esteem his work to be of importance. Here is a thought very pertinent to the desired attitude of the parent. *Let what your child does be important to you, and let him feel that you so consider it.* I know of nothing which so helps, inspires, and urges on a child— yes, a youth, or a man, or a woman—as does this feeling that the work in hand is really important to and appreciated by others. This may be accepted as a precept not only for parents but, also, for husbands and wives, and for brothers and sisters. If we can make another feel that his work is important to us, it promptly becomes important to him, and his effort becomes doubled, and happier, and better. Do not condole with your children because of their lessons! Do not say, "My! I am glad I don't have to study that!" Do not say, "I think your teacher is awful to ask so much." Do not say, "Never mind, this horrid school will soon be over—vacation will soon be here." Do not even tell them that you have forgotten all that you ever learned in school—keep that a secret; they may admire you, and if school knowledge is of no use to you, why then, they will reason, it certainly can be of no use to them. Children are often far more logical than they are given credit for. Their brain patterns are few, and their judgments are, therefore, generally wrong, but they frequently use the patterns they do possess, to the best possible advantage. To the child all this means, simply, "My studies are of no importance; they are merely something unpleasant and silly, an infliction of childhood, which must be lived through as best one may." What a fine incentive to study is this! Here is the teacher at school doing his or her best to rouse some sense of interest within the child, and here are the parents at home doing their best to negative the teacher's endeavour. What chance has the teacher to win in such a contest? Practically none; for the parent's suggestions are in the direction of ease and indifference, and coincide most happily with the child's own inclinations.

Just one word more in regard to our educational attitude, one word as to what may be legitimately expected. Mental limitations are absolute. "Against stupidity the gods themselves are helpless." Our standard of expectation can not be that of attainment, as we can not know, positively, the child's capability. Our standard must be that very different one—the measure of effort. The child's effort can be seen, there is no uncertainty here. Let this be the basis of your judgment of his work, and let this be that which you shall try to direct. Never mind the results—you must take your child as God (or you) made him.

It should be noted, however, that this level beyond which, with ordinary incentive, your child can not go, does not represent the absolute limit referred to above. Under extraordinary stimulus he can go further. Then it is that we hear such remarks as, "I didn't know it was in him." Well, he did not know it either; it was the supreme stimulus which made the supreme achievement possible. Witness what our boys have done in France, and the surprise which they themselves have often felt at their own actions. This supreme achievement does not belong to everyday life—do not expect it. The normal range of action is much lower. A man can not walk on tiptoe all the time. It is interesting, however, as revealing, in an exaggerated form, the potency of the adequate stimulus. It is interesting, also, as a final reminder that if your child fails it is yourself you should question—before you question him.

As to education in its relation to social reform, it is worth while to note that it can in no sense be regarded as a panacea. One man, *A*, may gain by education, but his superior, *B*, will gain more. In the end they retain their relative positions; *B* will still lead, and *A* will still be discontented with his lot. As a matter of fact, equallizing of opportunity in itself tends to accentuate differences, for under like conditions the superior man will always gain more than will the inferior, and will, therefore, always remain an object of envy. It is not lack of absolute possession that makes a man unhappy, it is seeing how much more the other fellow has gained. One finds no superior men in the army of the discontented. The good of ordinary education, then, is in its benefit to the state, in the raising of the general social level. It has little bearing upon the happiness of the individual. This again throws us back to what has been so often said, that *the education worth while for the individual is that which concerns itself with his habits and attitudes.* All roads in psychology lead to this same goal.

CHAPTER X

Its Nature and Contents

IT is evident that at any one time we are using but a small portion of our available brain patterns. Only a small part of our mental store can be before us at any one moment of our existence. It is as with our eye vision, we see clearly only that upon which we focus. From this central point vision fades toward the margin where lie but the vaguest suggestions of sight, and here, at the margin, it finally ends. Beyond the margin, however, there lies, we know, a vast world not now seen at all, but which, piecemeal, can be brought into vision by changing the direction of our gaze. In our mental field, likewise, we see only that upon which we focus, that to which we give our attention. Beyond this appreciated field of our present consciousness lies the vastly greater field of unconsciousness, the field of the subconscious mind, where lie all the hundreds of thousands of experiences, brain patterns, and emotional potentialities which constitute our inheritance and our experience in life. "There are secret and individual parts in the nature of men, and mute conditions without show, sometimes unknown of their very possessors." *

But let us go a step further—our unseen world is not a dead world awaiting our regard before it awakens. It is with the mentally unseen world of the subconscious mind as it is with the vast world unseen by our eyes. This subconscious, unconscious mind of ours is by no means the quiet storehouse it was once assumed to be—deep down in the unconscious mind things happen. It is a storehouse, it is true, but not one of mere inactive waiting. There is going on in the unconscious mind, though possibly in modified form, the very same processes that are known to our consciousness. An unconscious cerebration is there taking place, a modified activity corresponding in kind to that we have already studied. We store away experiences, but these do not necessarily, nor generally, remain isolated; they may, under certain conditions, form unconscious associations and undergo change, and when again brought to

* Montaigne.

consciousness may be altered beyond recognition. To the old orthodox attitude the above is absurd. In the old conception, with soul-controlled thought, the unconscious is simply something which is not. The poets and philosophers knew better. To them the unconscious has always been very real indeed, and so it is to the psychologists of today. The unconscious, it is believed, differs from the conscious merely in not being in focus, and in being incomparably greater and richer.

We must add one concept more, namely this: that from the unconscious excursions take place into the conscious and have an effect on our conscious lives—that there is, in fact, a two-way connection between the conscious and the unconscious, a connection by no means always under the control of the will. Take a very simple example of this. You are seeking a name; you can not recall it; you finally abandon the quest and turn to something else. Suddenly the name comes to you—bobs up, as it were, from the unconscious into the conscious. While *you* were thinking of something else, the original mental process was continued in the unconscious, and there finally found the pattern sought. Or, more elaborately, we are striving to solve a problem, and can not, and give it up, and go to bed—and then wake in the morning with the answer clearly before us.*

Does not this unconscious cerebration, which, it would seem, must be accepted, endorse the description of thought given earlier? Our picture then was of a nerve force, the neurokyme, which once set in action flowed here and there until it found the brain pattern which would solve the problem presented.

The fact that the unconscious sometimes succeeds better than our conscious effort is explainable, probably, by the presence in the latter of a wilful control which may be mistaken. Our conscious effort may be in the wrong direction, but we, nevertheless, obstinately hold to the path on which we have started. For example; we are trying to recall the name of a man, and we feel sure that it begins with a *B;* so we keep harping on Brown, and Baker, and Bissel, and Black—hanging on to the *B* idea at all costs. But when we finally give over the search, the *B* idea gets dropped also, and the subconscious, left to work it out by itself, finally finds what we want—the man's

---

* "We sleep, but the loom of life never stops; and the pattern which was weaving when the sun went down is weaving when it comes up tomorrow." This from Henry Ward Beecher! Though we must acknowledge that what he had in mind was quite other than the psycho-physiological phenomenon we are considering.

name was Adams. We remember now that we met him in Boston, and that is, of course, where the *B* idea came from.

These are examples of simple unconscious cerebration, and of recovery from the unconscious of facts lying, as it were, just beneath the surface. But this subconscious, unconscious region contains many, many other things than these temporarily laid aside items. In the unconscious lie all the memories, impressions, and experiences of life; events of our childhood, things near, and far past; things we have put away until needed; things we have tried to forget, and things we have forgotten. Here, too, are things we do not know and may never know we possess—passing impressions which may never have registered in the conscious mind, but which were, nevertheless, duly registered in the unconscious. Here, too, are our inheritances, our innate dispositions, our tendencies; some of them recognized by us at times; and some of them still but potentialities, their patterns never yet having been used, they never yet having received the stimulus necessary to set them in action. These last, we shall find, are important, for whether chance ever discovers them or not, they are there, and do surely affect, albeit unconsciously, our thoughts and our actions. Furthermore, being unsuspected, their control is neither sought nor obtained.

We have reached now to a conception of a vast region of unconscious cerebration, from which arise impulses and influences which, whether they actually come to consciousness or not, do, still, profoundly affect our conscious lives. From this seething underworld of thought come many of the inhibitions, or *stops,* which obstruct our conscious acceptances, and from it, too, come many of our calls to action. We are influenced we know not, consciously, how nor why; and we wonder at ourselves—it is the unconscious that is pulling!

This conception of the unconscious is not new, it is only the precise statement of it which is new. The poets have known it for ages, it is in this their truth lies; and the philosophers, with poetical minds, the only true philosophers, have endeavoured to express it in words. Philosophy, says Montaigne, is but a form of "sophisticated poesie." Listen to Philosopher Browning:

"So works Mind—by stress
Of faculty, with loose facts, more or less,
Builds up our solid knowledge: all the same,
Underneath rolls what Mind may hide not tame,

162

THE SUBCONSCIOUS MIND

An element which works beyond our guess,
Soul, the unsounded sea—whose lift of surge,
Spite of all superstructure lets emerge,
In flower and foam, Feeling from out the deeps
Mind arrogates no mastery upon. . . ."

When the modern conception of the unconscious is first brought to our attention, there always arises this question—are we then, in fact, its slaves? No, most certainly not! For while we can not alter the unconscious within us, nor ignore its impulses and influences, we can learn to control these impulses, and make them subserve to useful ends. Browning notwithstanding, mind may arrogate some mastery over that which comes "from out the deeps."

Here is the essence of the moral life—the drawing from this reservoir of good and bad, just that which is good. Here, indeed, lies the very reason for education, and here, also, the necessity for psychological knowledge on the part of the teacher. It is the understanding of the subconscious impulse which goes far to making a fascinating science of teaching. When a child won't learn, is stubborn and forgetful, or when he is eccentric and nervous, or wilful, the cause may easily lie in the unconscious mind, and, if understood, may be removable. Education is an effort at subconscious control, it aims at the mastery of the unconscious impulse. Or, to put it another way, education consists in the bringing out from the subconscious only that which is desirable and useful. Do not ask your child why he did so and so. He does not know—but *you* should! What is your child to be? He can not develop all of his inherited tendencies. He is descended from two parents, from four grandparents, and from eight great grandparents; in the tenth generation there were one thousand and twenty-four ancestors, and from that generation to this he has had, inclusive, two thousand and forty-six. The guidance you owe him, in selecting his path in life, is education—and this consists, as we have just seen, in the development of the conscious control of his unconscious possessions, quite as much as it does in the forming for him of new brain patterns.

The Mind Cure

If we will recognize the influence of the conscious on the unconscious mind, as stated in the last section, the question then rises—why should not the conscious mind also influence the unconscious act? We have conscious thoughts and conscious acts, and we have un-

conscious thoughts and unconscious acts—are
not these all necessarily connected? Conscious
thought naturally results in conscious act, but
we have just found that it also influences the unconscious thought—why not, then, through this,
the unconscious act?

What do we mean by unconscious acts?
They are many, especially those which we call
physiological—those activities of the body by
which, quite unconsciously to ourselves, life is
maintained. Here we have the heart beat, the
respiration, the digestion, and the glandular
functions; and here we have all the thousands
of chemical and physical reactions going on in
the microscopic cells of our bodies—reactions
which together make up the life of the body.
Remembering that good health depends upon
these physiological acts being carried out in the
best possible manner, and that ill health results
when they are improperly performed, it becomes evident that in considering the influence
of the conscious mind on the unconscious act,
we are, in reality, considering that old question,
the influence of mind over matter—and now
especially in its physiological application, the
mind cure.

Fortunately we do not have to use a theoretical approach to the subject; there is no room

for argument; the experience is universal. We *know* that our conscious thoughts and our conscious mental attitudes do affect at least some of these unconscious physiological acts, and if it be denied that they also affect others, the burden of proof falls naturally on the denier. We know that certain thoughts will increase respiration and heart beat, and that certain others will retard these same acts. We know that happy thoughts favour digestion, and that unhappiness and worry impede it. We know, experimentally, that oxidation changes within the blood and tissues are modified by the conscious emotional state, and, this being so, we have reason to believe that all those more subtile and multitudinous chemical and physical reactions which go to make up life must be also affected. But these circulatory and other subtile reactions are, we know, what determine our health. The inference is unavoidable—health must be largely influenced by the mental attitude, and a change from an unhealthful to a healthful attitude must tend toward cure when disease already exists.

We know little of all the intimate relations which must exist between the mind and the body, but certain of these we do know, and so important are they that based upon them alone there have been founded numerous cults of mental healing. I refer especially to the influence of fear and worry. The Christian Science cures, and the Menti-culture and miracle cures are all exhibitions of the influence I have claimed. These, and all other similar phenomena, whatever the jargon used, are based, in reality, upon the same scientific foundation. Christian Science is a fact, not a theory; and interest in it is common, whether this interest be expressed in sympathy or in scorn—the fact is that Christian Science gets results, and this outweighs all adverse criticism. We may resent the absurdities it preaches, but it can not be "poofed" aside. A saner and more satisfactory attitude toward it is to try to apprehend the underlying truth, and separate this from the error. I say the Christian Scientist gets results—he does, both good and bad. Sometimes he is a murderer, and sometimes a suicide; but then, again, sometimes he is a blessing—however much his disguise.

Let us turn for a moment to a consideration of *cure*. Most diseases tend to get well of themselves—there is a strong proclivity, in this our habit-formed body, to get back to a normal habit and rhythm—but conditions, of course, must be favourable. In most of our "cures" what we really do is to aid in making the conditions right—it is nature that does the curing. We know the value of good and proper hygiene, of good and appropriate food; also, of appropriate rest, or, it may be, exercise. These things being right, the body, unless profoundly disturbed, will generally manage to care for itself. The physician's part is to give to the public the benefit of his special knowledge of the conditions most conducive to health. He may depend entirely upon hygiene, or he may administer certain medicines which, in his experience, he knows will assist, or be needed to start, the restorative process. It may be that surgery will aid, or be necessary, but, even here, it is nature which will ultimately establish the cure —the surgeon merely removes some, maybe otherwise insuperable, obstacle.

Whether it be by aid of surgery, medicine, hygiene, or food, the cure is effected by obtaining the favouring body condition. Now, as has been suggested above, one factor remains to be considered; and it may be safely asserted that in the generality of cases, whatever the means used, no other is quite so singly important as is this—the mental attitude of the patient. That fear and worry, for example, make all improvement difficult, is a matter of common experience; and that cheerfulness and trust are helpful, we equally know. This is well recognized, and the physiological nature, even, of the influence is not now entirely unknown. The destructive emotion of fear has a direct influence on the adrenal and thyroid glands; substances are produced which, reaching the blood, if not at once used in flight or in fight, act as positive poisons. Fear has been described as an "unfled flight," or as a flight with the body in chains; the chemical state so produced is a toxic one, and most damaging to all healthful progress.

All this is recognized, but the practical application of it is generally missed. We know perfectly well that the mental attitude is important but we do not act on this knowledge; we leave action to charlatans. The average physician of today retains the old conventional attitude; he is willing to grant, conditionally, that the mind may have some effect in "nervous diseases," but he is not willing to concede any influence in the grosser physical disturbances. To this kind of a doctor there seems to be some mysterious difference between nerve cells and other cells. When the latter are affected it is an "organic disease"; when the former, why then it is "just nervous.'' It is this kind of a doctor, too, who is to be held responsible for these very cults he so much despises. Were the medical profession to recognize that mental influence which so many of the laity have discovered for themselves, there would be but little room for the fakir. Nervous diseases are not alone, nor even especially, susceptible to the mental influence. If the truth of what has gone before be granted, it is clear that this influence must extend equally to all of the physiological acts of the body, and must be ever a powerful agent both in keeping us well, and in the restoring to health when needs be. Do not misunderstand this statement. It does not say that a correct mental attitude must always result in cure; it says, simply, that the mental attitude is one of the most powerful single aids to cure, and that it is comparable with, but may even excel in importance, most of the other measures of hygiene.

So real is this influence that it operates even in extremity. Incurable diseases are notably relieved by a healthful mental attitude, and the effect may be obtained up to the very hour of death. The dying Roman Catholic, after receiving Extreme Unction, the last rite of the church, will often show, for a time, an improvement in condition—fear and worry as to the future having been replaced by gentle resignation and hope. On the other hand, when a very ill person gives up in despair, we know how quickly he will take a turn for the worse.

A bad mental attitude may easily negative all other means used to restore a patient to health. Hygiene, good food and medicine may all prove impotent; the mental attitude may be so bad that cure can not be effected. Then it is we hear of "the poor sufferer, who has been ill for years, whom the best physicians have been unable to relieve," suddenly getting well under Christian Science treatment, or, maybe, by a visit to Lourdes, or to Ste. Anne de Beau Prés. When the mental attitude was changed, cure came. In this sense, Christian Science has "cured" disease, as it has, also, prolonged life in incurable cases. It is a curious state of affairs, however, that the underlying scientific fact should be denied by the Christian Scientists, and the actual benefit ascribed to the inanities of an illogical creed. It is like putting on a life-preserver *and* a medal of some saint, and then, finding that one does not sink, accounting for this fact by the medal. The truth is, the scientific mind is not common even among well-educated people. Here is an

171

observed fact, Mrs. Eddy explains it—the fact is there, so Mrs. Eddy must be right! As has been said of one of their books, Christian Science contains much that is new, and much that is true; but that which is new is not true, and that which is true is not new. In its religious aspect it is an offence and an insult to reason, but underlying its "cure" is the scientific fact, we repeat it once more, that conscious mental attitudes do have an influence on the unconscious physiological functions of the body, and hence must affect the course of both life and disease. The essential atmosphere of cure is a state of happy confidence, and the process is the same whether this be given to a physician, to the teaching of Mary Mason Baker Patterson Glover Eddy, or to a bone from the toe of some saint.

I have just been reading an account of some cures by a man named Hickson. In these, as in all such, the true nature of the cure would seem to be apparent. One, who was paralyzed, can now wiggle his toes—but not yet walk. Another, who was blind, can now distinguish light and shadow—but not yet form. Are not such improvements just such as would be expected from an improved mental attitude? How can they be considered, by a Christian, to be the result of divine intervention? Can God's power give motion to a toe, but remain inadequate to completely restore health? Or is it that God has a scale of values for His services and that for so much faith He will give just so much cure? Such a god is not God the Creator, it is a little personal god, who stands ready, when sufficiently flattered by faith, to aid us to the best of his ability. The truth is, the improvement in the face of incurable disease, noted above, is the natural effect of a new and inspiring stimulus calling forth a fuller, happier, and more hopeful effort on the patient's part.

What is the useful moral of all this? Be brave! Be courageous! Men are not influenced by things, says Epictetus, but by their thoughts about things. Try to eliminate from these thoughts all fear, worry, and anger. To use a phrase of Horace Fletcher's, *emancipate* your bodies, and give them a chance. If you succeed you will be as well as any Christian Scientist, and you will, moreover, have preserved and increased, not abandoned, your intellectual self-respect.

It will be a matter of wonder to some that in treating of this subject I have said nothing of "suggestion," for with many it is this that

173

first comes to mind when mental influences in health are referred to. It is a well thrashed out subject—and it is precisely for this reason that I have preferred to dwell on a deeper and more fundamental relation. That suggestion plays a large part in many mind cures, can not be doubted; and especially is this true in the "nervous cases," where "suggestibility" is often so prominent a feature. But it may be doubted whether the cure by suggestion is often a permanent cure. The fact that suggestion operates at all is in itself evidence of a certain degree of mental instability; and the effect, therefore, generally soon wears off. In hysteria specific symptoms may thus be easily removed; but the disease itself remains unaltered, and only too often the symptom so removed is quickly replaced by another. Still, suggestion is subtile, and its influence is probably more frequent than most of us realize. Certainly good suggestions must accompany all successful efforts in mental cure, and, in the broadest sense, they most probably underlie all that with which we have just been dealing. It is in this broader aspect that I hold suggestion important; it is here but a step toward the attainment of the healthy mind.

THE SUBCONSCIOUS MIND

Mysticism

We have been considering the interplay between the conscious mind and the subconscious. Let us now consider what happens when the conscious control and conscious activities are lessened—either by deliberate intention, as in the voluntary contraction of the conscious field; or by a natural lowering, as in sickness, of that nerve force required for full conscious action. With the decrease of nerve force, the nerve voltage, the production of a vivid picture may become no longer possible; touch and pain, and conscious perceptions generally, may fail to attain to a normal reality. The individual sinks to a lower plane, where reverie and imagination become as real as that which is directly perceived. There comes a sense of loss of reality—a sensation familiar enough to, all who have suffered severe illness.

It is this condition which has given rise to mysticism; it is, in fact, this which is the mystic state—that seeing with closed eyes, as Plotinus has defined it. The threshold of consciousness, in the sense of wilful control, is lowered, and the subconscious pours in unimpeded. The perceptions of the conscious mind lose their normal strength; and portions of the subconscious, as in a waking dream, attain to the reality of the conscious. The individual can hardly distinguish between the two, and ends by not being able to distinguish at all; he floats in a world half real and half unreal, and he can not say which is which.

When this mystic state has been produced by loss of nerve energy, the feeling arrived at is generally one of insufficiency, of incompleteness, with, too, a sense of loss of the ego; but when the state is more or less a product of *will,* when the individual has deliberately contracted the conscious field, then the sense of insufficiency may be lacking and only the loss of ego remain. Self here seems gone, and, with the loss of finite control, there enters a sense of the infinite. Suppose now it happens that the individual who is experiencing this state has long been in the habit of concentrating upon Good, the life to come, and upon God—with the merging of the finite into the infinite, it is the finite self only which is lost, and he finds himself, or thinks himself, glorified by this very fact. Now at last, he feels, he has come in some mysterious way into contact with another world, with the world of infinity; and it may even be, through his loss of sense of self, that he will believe his soul to have actually entered into holy communion with the Godhead. This is religious mysticism—here are included all those mystic experiences which men here and there, of all races and climes and times, have shared in—Hindu, Buddhist, Mohammedan, and Christian.

The Hindu Yogi is a disciple of mysticism who by the mystic insight has attained to Samâdhi, the mystic of "superconscious" state. Let me quote from the Bhagavad-Gita: *

"The Saint who shuts outside his placid soul
All touch of sense, letting no contact through;
Whose quiet eyes gaze straight from fixéd brows,
Whose outward and inward breath are drawn
Equal and slow through nostrils still and close;
That one—with organs, heart, and mind constrained,
Bent on deliverance, having put away
Passion, and fear, and rage; hath, even now,
Obtained deliverance. . . ."

So the Buddhist, by concentrated contemplation, seeks to attain Dhyâna. He speaks of "elevated concentration," an intentness of meritorious thought, and finds it "noble, because it brings one into the possession of the magical powers and other blessings." In what is known as the Trance of Cessation, there are several stages corresponding to the degree of

* Translation by Sir Edwin Arnold.

contraction of the conscious mind. Starting with loss of desire, and of reason, one reaches, in the fifth and sixth stages, the true mystic state, described here as the realm of Infinity of Space, and the realm of Infinity of Consciousness. But the Buddhist goes on—the seventh stage is Nothingness, and the eighth is that of "Neither Perception nor yet Non-perception," and the ninth is Cessation itself, just short of death and Nirvana. Buddhism is a pessimistic religion—all flesh is bad, and the final good in life is a state of nothingness or less. There is a shedding of all earthly relations, a do-nothingness of *both* the conscious and the unconscious mind. The Christian mystic, on the other hand, abandons the conscious control only, and rests in the realms of infinity of space and of consciousness. He is carried upward in the rosy cloud of his dominant religious aspiration, and is brought to a nearness with God. All secrets are unlocked—the Trinity, the purposes of God, the Godhead itself, are all understood—but, alas! the experience remains an individual experience. The mystic *feels* but has no words with which to impart his knowledge.

Physiologically many of the extreme manifestations of mysticism are closely allied to hypnotism. The Buddhist priest, the Hindu Yogi, the Mohammedan Sufi, all use self-hypnotism, limiting, by practice, the conscious activities of the mind until they can at will attain that passive state of suggestibility which is characteristic of the hypnotized subject. For the hypnotic state is a passive state, a state where wilful control is abandoned, and the result is the same however this renunciation be accomplished, whether it be by outside suggestion, by "elevated contemplation," or by crystal gazing.

We know that, from the subconscious, impulses may and do rise into the conscious mind. In the ordinary course of events we give no heed to the origin of these impulses; they simply merge with the conscious thought. When however, they are particularly strong, or even when, as compared with the conscious activity, they are only relatively strong, they come to us with a distinct sense of strangeness, or outsideness, or, if one's mind runs in such a direction, of *inspiration*. If a man has a dominating, all controlling religious sentiment, and becomes conscious of the message from the subconscious, he has, he believes, been inspired by God. "The Word of God came to me," "God spake to me," "God spake to Moses," are expressions of these impulses, these inspirations. Here is the essence of revelation. Isaiah was so inspired—Mohammed, also. The Morman, today, is under this same guidance; the head of his church is the prophet, the seer, the revelator.

The prophets of the Hebrews were itinerant preachers; they were professionals, and they had followers who were students of their methods. They warned the people and the governors of the errors of their ways, and they spoke as men inspired. They *were* inspired—they were, in short, mystics, and spoke from that well of profound truth, the subconscious mind. The "bad prophets" were, maybe, those who were unable to obtain the true mystic insight, and who pretended and imitated only. To the former we owe much—above all, our conception of a spiritual God. The ancient Yahweh, the national deity of the early Hebrew people, became, through the prophets' teaching, Elohim, or God as we conceive God, an omnipresent, omniscient, infinite, spiritual power.

The Yahweh of the early Hebrews was a national god; there was no idea, even with them, of his being the only God. Other nations had their own gods, but Yahweh was the Hebrew's god, or, rather, they were Yahweh's chosen people. He was their monarch, they were his subjects. He was a jealous god, an angry god, a vengeful god. "I am Jehovah, thy God, who brought thee out of the Land of Egypt, out of the house of bondage. Thou shalt have no other gods, before me." Here was a god who must be placated with sacrifice and ceremony, or he would crush the delinquent.

Now mysticism, which I have spoken of as the valuable root of the prophets' teachings, does not lead to any such anthropomorphic conception as this. It does not lead to a man god, but to a sense of infinity, to a sense of a limitless spiritual essence; to a feeling concept, not to an intellectual one—this last can only be finite. It was this feeling, this sense of an infinite presence, that the prophets brought to the Hebrew people. To it was given the name Elohim—God —and now, for the first time, the Hebrews became truly monotheistic, and entered upon that extension of belief which has made their religion the background of our world-wide Christianity. This is what we owe to the mysticism of the Hebrew prophets—who came down, like Christ, out of the north, into Judea.

Spiritualism and Telepathy *

Mysticism, as we have seen, implies a lessening of the conscious control, with incursions of impulses from the unconscious into the conscious field. But these impulses may also reach consciousness without any such preliminary loss of control and without, therefore, producing that sense of the infinite upon which mysticism depends. In this second type of case the sense of inspiration remains, but the experience is interpreted as "psychic" rather than as divine. The sense is of the supernatural, and spiritual, but not of infinity, for the ego is retained and contact still held with the finite. Two worlds are now sensed as co-existing in time—the finite world of the conscious mind, and the supernatural, an outside world, also finite, of the spirit.

The experience is common, more common than is that of the mystic state, and spiritualism, its product, is a matter of faith to the many. We are dealing here with a phenomenon as old as man, with a faculty of the mind which has

* In using the title "spiritualism" to cover all of that which follows, I bow to custom, though, personally, I would prefer to observe the distinction made by Flournoy : " We must not confound *spiritism,* which is a pretended scientific explanation of certain facts by the intervention of spirits of the dead, with *spiritualism,* which is a religio-philosophical belief." From translation by H. Carrington.

doubtless existed since the conscious activity of
mind began. Nor is the belief in spiritualism
likely ever to die away; the inter-relation of the
subconscious and the conscious must always
persist, and it is hardly to be expected but that
this relation shall ever remain more or less of a
mystery to the masses. More than this—behind the faith there lies that powerful determinant, the Will to Believe; a force so potent that
the intellect itself bows before it. Spiritualism
is an answer to man's most urgent interroga-
tions, the *what* and *how* of the future, and as
such it has swayed, and will sway, the minds of
educated and ignorant alike.

Looking at it from a slightly different angle,
spiritualism is a response to a craving for sim-
plification of thought; and it is curious to remark that the man of science is after this very
same thing. Belief in and denial of spiritualism, in the last analysis, rest on the same inherent demand of our minds. What the one
explains by spiritism, the other explains by his
materialistic monism, and, psychologically,
neither can claim an advantage. Monism, as
was said in the chapter on Thought, is a useful hypothesis but can in no sense be regarded
as a demonstrated fact. The best that can be
said for it is that it is nearer in form to other

scientific findings than is the non-materialistic conception of the spiritist.

Why is it that spiritualism is so especially in the thought of the world today? The answer, I believe, is obvious, but let us put it in words.

Death is a reality, accepted as such, and appreciated in a way, under certain conditions. As the end of a gradual dissolution, in old age; or as the end of an illness where suffering and pain have long been inmates of the home, when patient and attendants have become mentally and physically fatigued and the idea of death has long hovered in the thought—then death comes, and is accepted. There follows, the funeral and the grave. Our beloved one is gone; we have bade him goodbye; we have seen him depart; this is the end so far as this life is concerned. We accept, and turn now for consolation to those teachings of the next world to which we have been born, or in which, in times of calmer thought, we have learned to believe.

But in war time, or in the blank aftermath of war, how different the situation! Here is Youth in fine vigour, full of ambition and worldly loves, and Youth marches away amid plaudits of enthusiastic encouragement; marches away, writes jolly letters home, and then—the letters cease. Is there any reality in death, here? Such a death is incredible; this living dynamo of immortal youth *must* be alive; he can not be dead. We can not accept so vacant a thought. He is gone "over there"— and he must still be "over there," or somewhere, in all his same happy vitality.

As an intellectual concept we do, of course, admit the death, but our feelings do not join our intellect in this supine acceptance. This youth must be alive even though he has, they say, departed this life. We know he must be somewhere, and we feel sure, even, that he will communicate with us if he can. The spiritualist says that he *is here,* that he is struggling to communicate with us—surely the spiritualist is right! I feel that what he says is true— don't talk to me of a vague, unknowable Heaven—this veil my boy has passed through does not open upon any such abstraction! As a living spirit, here, in this world—yes, I can accept that, and I can enjoy and rest in this sweet thought. I thank God for opening my eyes!

To this, as a "religio-philosophical belief," there can be no scientific objection; but as to the phenomena which are supposed to endorse it, there is much to be said.

Let us consider this matter. We know that

impulses pass from the unconscious mind to the conscious; and we know that these impulses, if strong, carry with them a sense of outsideness, of strangeness. These we have already considered from the standpoint of inspiration, and we know how real they have been, and are, as influences in the life of man. The prophets were so inspired, and so have we all been in some humble degree. It is the strength of the impulse, not its existence, that brings in the sense of the supernatural.

Now what is true of wordless impulses and of ideas, so originating in the subconscious mind, is equally and more simply true of other mental reactions. Let the auditory area be sufficiently stimulated, and we *hear;* let the visual area be so stimulated, and we *see;* it does not matter whence the stimulation comes, whether over the usual afferent nerves of hearing and seeing, or whether entirely of internal origin. In the first case, however, we call the "affect" a perception, while in the latter we call it an hallucination. In the hallucination, then, the image is produced by internal stimulation and has no connection with the external world. Why then is it regarded as coming from outside? As well ask why any true perception is so regarded. For consider again what has

186

just been said—vision and hearing are due to stimulation, but it is the stimulation itself that is important, not its origin. Light does not pass over the optic nerve to the visual centre in the brain, a stimulus only so passes, a nerve impulse which excites certain brain cells to action. What we see is really all within our own heads; it is merely our interpretation of the action of the brain cells. And the same is true of all we hear, smell, taste, and feel—the perception is a mental process, the result of the activity of certain cells, *regardless of the cause of that activity*. There are brain diseases in which the patients are tormented by vile odours; and there are others where voices, and sounds, and sensations annoy—all external in seeming, but all actually of internal origin.

It is largely experience which establishes the normal projection of our perceptions into their proper position in space; we learn by experience to locate the cause of our visions and other impressions as external to ourselves. Once established, however, the same judgment is habitually continued even when false. A rough parallel is found in the fact that a man may lose a leg by amputation, and suffer long after from pains in the foot that is gone, and the pains in this "phantom limb" may be quite as real as though the limb was still there.

Stimulation, then, of a visual area, even when the stimulation is from within, will result in a mental picture which, *if the stimulation be sufficiently vivid,* will be interpreted as though it came, as normally, from an external source. Less vivid stimulation will result in a memory only. When we recall the appearance of the outside of the building we are in, we excite, though only mildly, certain brain cells to action. Let these same cells be sufficiently stimulated and we would *see* the building. This vivid internal stimulation we can not accomplish by will, but it frequently occurs in disease. When in the excitement of a fever we become delirious, we see, hear, and live in a life entirely mental, but very real for us. Our world then is a world of abnormally stimulated brain patterns; the psychogenic force is lowered; the conscious field is contracted; and the subconscious mind, stimulated by the toxins of the disease and by circulatory changes, comes strongly into play. The sensation is very different from that obtained by the mild, partial stimulation of memory. Delirium may be described as a turbulent action of the subconscious mind, a vivid stimulation with resulting images, uncensored by any conscious control. What has happened to most of us in fevers, others, the insane, experience daily.

The hallucinations, illusions, and delusions of the fever patient, and of the insane, differ in no way, so far as their origin is concerned, from those of the honest spiritist medium—supposing such to exist. The latter is, of course, neither ill nor insane, but he does share with both of these classes the tendency to vivid subconscious stimulation.

Practically all scientifically inclined spiritists, Lodge, *et al.*, willingly concede the natural agencies which have here been spoken of, and they even recognize the frequency of fraud, but they contend that neither natural law nor fraud can explain all the phenomena observed. They assume that the medium is unable to restrain himself from the playing of tricks,

"That's th' medium nature, thus they're made" *

and that he, like the rest of us, only more so, is subject to the vagaries of the subliminal mind. Nevertheless, mixed in with all this, they say, is an occasional, veritable, supernatural phenomenon. What the ultimate outcome of

* Browning: *Mr. Sludge, The Medium.* q.v. for the last word on this subject.

their researches may be, it is hard to say. Even if we should concede all that they claim, "when people come to understand that this sorting of messages [the true from the false] is almost beyond their power they will, perhaps, be put out of conceit with experiments in which they have ninety-nine chances against one of being duped, by themselves or others, and in which—a still more vexatious matter—if they should even be so fortunate as to light upon the hundredth chance, they would have no certain means of knowing it." *

Men of science have believed in spiritualism —they are welcome to their belief, but this, it should be recognized, has no real weight as an endorsement. Belief in spiritualism is an "over belief" such as any one is entitled to; it is not denied by science, but neither is it based upon any scientific foundation. To the psychologist, of course, it is interesting as a mental phenomenon, but to scientific men in general it is usually a matter of indifference so foreign it is, and so unpromising a field for research.

One elemental guiding rule in science is to accept no occult, supernatural explanation for that which can be satisfactorily and simply ex-

* Flournoy, in *From India to the Planet Mars.* See *Spiritism and Psychology.* Translated by H. Carrington.

plained by natural law. All "spiritual phenomena" may be so explained. There is nothing to suggest that there are any other processes involved in so-called spiritualism than those of known brain action. The seeing of spirits, the hearing of spirit voices, are simply manifestations of the subconscious mind—when not the result of a trick. The performances of the ouija board and automatic writing in general are, in the same way, motor performances done under subconscious control. When a scientific man comes to believe in spiritualism it is because he has, within a certain "reserved area" of his mind, yielded to his emotional inclination. Under the influence of the "will to believe" he has gradually dropped the critical attitude which belongs to science; and he has arrived where he is, not by applying scientific methods, as he often claims, but by abandoning them. As has been said, he is welcome to his belief—if he will but drop his cant concerning science. There is nothing in spiritualism which may not be true—it is simply not proven, nor even scientifically suggested. Reason must be limited to that which can be demonstrated; what lies beyond, reason should neither deny nor endorse.

When we recall the strangeness of many of

the psychic phenomena, they may seem a heavy burden to place upon the subconscious mind, but let us turn back to the first section of this chapter and consider again the nature of the subconscious contents. There will be found many strange things—"things unknown of their very possessors."

Let me give one example, an old, but a good one. A young, illiterate, peasant woman, during the crisis of a nervous breakdown, recited fluently in Latin, in Greek, and in Hebrew. After long inquiry it was finally ascertained that she had once served as a servant for a learned pastor whose custom it was to walk up and down, in a passage way of his house, reading aloud from his favourite authors. It was these fragmentary phrases, floating in through the open kitchen door, which the girl, without the faintest understanding, had received and registered in her unconscious mind. How eagerly the Society for Psychical Research would have welcomed this wonder! Fortunately she happened to be a hospital case.

I have said that all the experiences of spiritualism are easily explained by science. There are, however, certain allied manifestations to which science can give no entirely satisfactory explanation. I refer to telepathy, and

to thought transmission in its varied forms of
clairvoyance, somnambulism, and mental suggestion. Whether we are, or are not, here in the
presence of an unknown force, I do not know.
The evidence is extremely difficult to value, and
the judicial attitude very difficult to maintain.
Those who "account for" psychical phenomena
simply by denying their existence, do so with
vehemence—with a vehemence derived from
their dislike of the supernatural—but this
vehemence is, in itself, also, evidence of their
own unscientific prejudice. Why bring in the
supernatural at all? Is it not possible that we
may be here in face with a natural law as yet
undiscovered, a natural force as yet only partially recognized? It would certainly be unscientific and presumptious to deny the possibility that such a force may exist. To deny its
possibility would be to seat ourselves with Gali-
leo's judges.*

We know many things in nature very imper-
fectly, and of causes we know practically nothing. It may thus easily be, as Flammarion long
ago has claimed, that there is existing a
"psychic force" known to us, so far, only by

* To quote from the heading of a chapter by Flammarion, "On
Incredulity."
  "Croire tout decouvert est une erreur profonde
  C'est prendre l'horizon pour les bornes du monde."
                                          LAMARTINE.

its occasional results—an unknown force emanating from the human being, and capable of making itself felt at a distance. This possibility we will concede, but let us be on our guard—the possibility of an unknown force is in no way evidence that such a force exists. Such a conclusion would be as illogical as is that of Sir Oliver Lodge, who argues that because science presents marvels to the uninitiated layman therefore spiritualism ought to be believed in.

Inexplicable phenomena are common—why? For two reasons: either we do not have all the facts necessary for the explanation, or the phenomenon is produced according to laws not yet discovered. Into which of these categories telepathy is to be placed will depend on the bias of the reader. We can all recite numerous interesting experiences, some of them, maybe, at first hand. My mother came down to breakfast one morning announcing that her brother, of whom she had had no recent knowledge, was, she knew, in great trouble. Before breakfast was ended we received a telegram telling of the brother's sudden death during the night. Again, while I was studying medicine in Edinburgh, a similar presentiment had led her to have my father cable for information as to my health. The "very day and hour" my mother had her presentiment of trouble, I was—in perfect health and contentment, and so continued. A certain philosopher, on being shown the thanks-offerings in a temple to Neptune, inquired, "Where are those commemorated who never came back?" The fact is, in things of this kind, as Bacon says—men mark when they hit, not when they miss.

Fortuitous coincidence is doubtless accountable for many of the telepathic phenomena. One distinguished psychologist, as the result of thousands of experiments, has decided that telepathic "successes" do not exceed that which might be expected from the mathematical principles of chance. It would seem, however, that this investigator has proved too much. For what is chance? It is certainly not always what the mathematician means by the term. What we call chance in life is often the definite result of unrealized causes. This being so, results in telepathy should exceed the mathematical expectation, for many of the successes there are doubtless due not to true chance but to causes which may be ordinary enough, though hidden and unnoticed.

There are undoubtedly simple explanations for much that at first seems strange. A premonitory dream, for instance, at first thought seems impossible of scientific explanation—but is it? May it not be, after all, simply a shrewd estimate of that which may happen, the result of a subconscious inductive process?

Let me illustrate by taking examples from everyday life. These will not be interesting, but they are important because it is largely upon such personal experiences that our readiness to believe in the more remarkable is based.

You have not heard from nor thought of a certain friend for a long time; he comes to your mind, and you sit down and write to him; he does the same by you, and the letters cross. Now the cause of this mutual thought may be simple enough. It may be a season of the year with some mutual association; the time of some former trip together, or of an important meeting. It may be a month in which something once happened of mutual interest; or some common friend may have recently died, or married, or eloped. It may be that some event has been recorded in the newspapers which you know would interest your friend—he sees the same, and knows that it would interest you. Or it may be any one of a hundred things which have a sufficient content of common interest to turn one's thought to the other. Note, too, that

196

the connecting link may have been *unconsciously* registered in the mind—in none of these cases need there be the slightest conscious recognition of their suggestive nature; the appreciation of the suggestion may remain entirely subconscious.

Again, you are in a department store and you suddenly come face to face with a friend, and you exclaim, "Isn't it funny? I was just thinking of you." What may have happened is that you have already seen your friend, and did not know it. You have passed her standing, maybe, at a counter; and you have caught, quite unconsciously, a glimpse of her—but only a glimpse, not sufficient to register a recognition in the conscious mind, though quite sufficient to produce a subconscious registration, and thus start a train of thought. Cryptopsychism is the term which has been suggested to cover these hidden, unobserved perceptions and memories, which, though unregistered consciously, still govern our actions.

Now these cryptopsychic experiences are often called telepathic, and, as I have said, they truly do prepare our minds for belief in telepathy in general. On the other hand, if these have an ordinary explanation, is it not possible that the more remarkable psychic phenomena may have the same—if only the facts could be known?

There is one feature of this question which remains to be spoken of, namely, the difficulty in obtaining true testimony. In all honest efforts to record telepathic and spiritual experiences great stress is placed upon the credibility of the witness. But the fact is that *no witness is entirely credible*. The best intentioned, neutral witness will make many mistakes, and when the witness is not neutral, when he has a bias, even though he still be well intentioned, he will make many more. This is not pleasant, but it is true. Many tests have been made along this line, and always with remarkable uniformity of result. Professor Swift says: "Experiments have proved that, in general, when the average man reports events or conversations from memory, and conscientiously believes that he is telling the truth, about one-fourth of his statements are incorrect." Münsterberg reports a test in which leading men of affairs took part. A simple episode was enacted in a broker's office; there were but four actors, and the entire incident occupied but a few moments of time. Not one of the twenty lawyers and bankers present was able afterwards to describe, in its essentials, what had actually taken place. The majority made from fifty to sixty per cent of omissions, and substituted so many false details, that in many of the reports a third of the description was contrary to fact. It is a pity that we can not return to the old Roman custom, which prefaced all testimony with the phrase, " It seemeth unto me."

The reasons for this, so important, peculiarity or weakness of mankind, may be gathered from our earlier chapters—we may recite them, again briefly, as follows: emotion and bias, uncertainties of perception, the influence of the will to believe, the power of suggestion, *hindthought and elaboration to fit it, and the imaginative filling of expected details.* When we come to the recounting of experiences in spiritualism and telepathy, these influences will be found to be specially active. The truth is that most people who retail spiritual and telepathic experiences believe in them, and want you to believe in them; their stories lose nothing in the telling—indeed they improve; weak points discovered in one recital are corrected or eliminated in the next. It is human nature; the intention is not necessarily dishonest. The teller of marvels wants his audience to experience what he has experienced, so if his first telling does not produce the desired thrill, the next time he tells it he improves it. He falsifies it to make it more true.

Briefly then, in summary, the position of the man of science is that, while there is no scientific reason to deny spiritualism, it is unnecessary, and unprofitable, and unreasonable, to seek for supernatural causes for that which known laws are adequate to explain. This he believes to be the case with all the so-called spiritual phenomena. The visions, the voices, the sense of presence, all follow known laws governing the action of the human mind. It is man's desire for an after-world within his comprehension; it is his desire to remain in contact, even if only spiritually, with a finite world—this is what gives rise to belief in spiritualism—this, and the fact that the impulses from the subconscious mind must always remain strange and inexplicable to the uninitiated. As regards telepathy, we grant that there may be a natural psychic force, as yet unknown, but we reserve our opinion. Very little evidence of sufficient scientific value to warrant study has as yet been presented; and when sufficient data have been obtained, the so-called psychic experience has invariably proven either a fraud, or the product of an already known law. However, credulity and incredulity are equally vicious;

the scientific mean should be of a sort of judicious diffidence.

No attempt has been mǎde to correlate and describe all the "psychic phenomena." They are multiform, but, nevertheless, all are fairly well grouped under the two heads given, the spiritual, and the telepathic. And these, too, are intimately related, for telepathy has been used to explain spiritualism, and spiritualism has been used to explain telepathy. Hypnotism, of course, plays a large and important part, especially in the spiritist séance.

One complication should be mentioned, in closing, and that is the possible presence of mental disease. Belief in spiritualism undergoes remarkable exaggerations when combined with paranoia, and other mental derangements; and churches, even, have been founded by these victims of delusion.

Truth and the Subconscious Impulse

To thousands of mystics, the world over, the mystic world is the true world, and that which we know only in the normal consciousness is the artificial and limited world, and something to be rid of. Even where there is no such extreme belief, the opinions which originate in the subconscious, the result of subconscious incubation, are the opinions we most cherish, no matter how foolish they may be. They are the ones we believe in most, while those which have purely intellectual value have really but little weight in our decisions. We must feel, as well as know, before we are convinced. Thus, I *know*, intellectually, that one of the chief causes for the high cost of living is in the inflation of the currency, but I have nothing in my subconscious inheritances to make me *feel* this fact, and it therefore remains to me of but little force—I forget it constantly, and seek some other, more emotional, cause.

We tend to hold on to these subconscious ideas as something belonging peculiarly to ourselves, as part of self, and we maintain them even against our own criticism. The reason for this is that measuring very large in the subconscious are the innate dispositions, our inheritances from the past; and here, too, lie all our subconscious acceptances of the mores, our group customs, as well as our earliest acquired habits. Now innate dispositions, feelings and emotions, temperamentally influenced, and adjusted to our mores, constitute the very essence of self. All so founded must necessarily command our utmost respect—these are the things which are *true* for us.

And yet, often the overcoming of an innate tendency gives us a very special sense of satisfaction, and of pride in our ego. How is this, if our real ego is that which exists in the unconscious mind, and itself includes the innate tendencies? The explanation of this seeming contradiction lies in the fact that it is not the conscious mind alone which has established the victory, but rather the self-regarding sentiment, which, itself, has its roots deep in the unconscious. What has happened is that the self-regarding sentiment has condemned this certain innate tendency, has judged it to be alien to its conception of the whole, and has, with all the strength of both its conscious and unconscious elements, determined to eliminate it. The satisfaction arising from this renunciation, successfully carried out, is due to the greater harmony of the mental complexes remaining; and follows the general rule that the physiological pleasure of a completed act is always in proportion to the absence of conflicting desires and impulses.

"Truth is within ourselves; it takes no rise
From outward things, what e'er you may believe.
There is an inmost centre in us all,
Where truth abides in fulness; and around,

Wall upon wall, the gross flesh hems it in,
This perfect, clear perception—which is truth.

. . . And to know
Rather consists in opening out a way
Whence the imprisoned splendour may escape,
Than in effecting entry for a light
Supposed to be without. Watch narrowly
The demonstration of a truth, its birth,
And you trace back the effluence to its spring
And source within us; where broods radiance vast,
To be elicited ray by ray, as chance
Shall favour: . . ."

BROWNING: Paracelsus.

It is a strange fact that while the subconscious
emotional complex so largely determines our
thought, maintaining itself against all the as-
saults of cold reason, we nevertheless do not
like to be reminded of this control. While we
really *feel* our decisions, we like to consider
them as having been reached by purely intellectual processes. We dignify thought in our
minds at the expense of our feeling, though we
actually follow the latter and find it, only, true.
We feel a thing, and believe it, and then try to
find a reason for our belief, a thought to explain it—and then we say we have believed it
because of this thought! It is the same with

our actions. Listen to a boy trying to give a reason for some act he desires to perform. Consider the cant about going to war "to make the world safe for democracy"!

It is the subconscious feeling which fixes the truth for us of any proposition worth caring about—in others, more trivial, we let reason decide. No wonder, then, faith is unassailable, for faith is of the subconscious mind. The subconscious mind is the *heart*, in our manner of speech—that which is felt in the heart, that which comes from the heart. This unconscious hidden part of us, which we have so generally disregarded in favour of its modern off-shoot the conscious mind, is really our most cherished possession.

I trust that, in tracing the source of faith, and of spiritual aspirations generally, to the subconscious mind, I shall not seem to you to be robbing these great life forces of their value. That they are great forces, that they are worthy determinants of man's best conduct, is a matter of experience requiring no proof. As an example in parallel, the historical criticism of the Bible has taken away nothing but the conception of its supernatural writing; it has not taken away belief in the Bible as a source of consolation and guidance. As one devout Christian recently wrote, but a short time preceding his death, the Biblical criticism in removing "the burdensome obligation of attempting to defend as errorless everything found in the Bible . . . [has set man] free to concentrate his attention upon its spiritual appeal." *

So, in seeking the roots of spiritual force within our own minds, we should not feel that we are in any way lowering this force, as some have asserted, to a mere mechanical product of material origin. It may be that the power of God has chosen just this point of entrance into our lives; and that, as James has suggested, this subconscious continuance of our conscious mind may be really but the hither side of a vast unrevealed world of unknown force. Neither conscious effort, nor unconscious, can attain to the ultimate truth of life. "We are born to seek after truth—to possess it belongs to a greater power."

"The ladder lent
To climb by, step and step, until we reach
The little foothold-rise allowed mankind
To mount on and thence guess the sun's survey—
Shall this avail to show us world-wide truth?"

BROWNING.

* The late Howard S. Bliss, D.D., formerly head of the Protestant Syrian College of Beirut. The quotation is from the *Atlantic Monthly,* for May, 1920.

THE SUBCONSCIOUS MIND

Life is like the passage of a bird through a lighted room. Flying in from the darkness, it abides a moment, and then vanishes into the night whence it came. So said, once, a Saxon thane to his king, and, today, from the standpoint of knowledge, we have nothing to add. What may lie on the far side of the subconscious, we do not know, but, personally, I believe it to be real.

CHAPTER XI

Abnormality

ABNORMALITY, as regards the *individual*, consists in any departure, in mental state or reaction, from that average which is found in the mass of society. It includes such varying types as the idiot, the imbecile, the man of affairs, the genius, the diseased and physically deficient, and the insane. From the *social* standpoint, the abnormal is one who is unable, or unwilling, to adapt himself to the society in which he lives. He is one who has failed to make the required social adjustment; who is, in a word, socially inadequate. The classes here are as with the individual, though men of genius, inventors and originators—men of supermentality—might be better and more practically described as socially unusual, rather than as abnormal. If not amenable to all the social conventions, they are, at least, to the social necessities.

In this review the mental causes of abnormality will alone be considered, and, of these, especially the border-states, those nearest to the normal. Here we shall find the greatest practical problems.

We say of a man that he is eccentric and queer—what do we mean? Well, we may mean any of a hundred things. He may be deficient in brain development, and consequently prone to childish decisions. He may have an illy balanced inheritance of emotional reactions, or he may be lacking in some of these same; or he may have but slight power of fusing his emotions, and thus be always "flying to extremes." He may have the reverse of all this; he may have an exceptionally large number of associations, and, therefore, be unduly imaginative. His emotional inheritances may be excessively strong, either in part or in whole; or his emotions may fuse, but in unusual ways. This is merely touching on the possibilities—the nerve responses may be uncommonly quick, or uncommonly slow; the sentiments may be peculiar, too all-embracing, or too narrow, or illy balanced and conflicting. Other variations will make for the more desirable attributes. In short there are endless varieties, and to call a man abnormal does not specify him at all, it merely places him as a member of a very large class, and leaves his real nature still undetermined.

"Abnormal tendencies of mind are dispositions toward extreme or irregular functioning, marked enough to appear in the ordinary run to situations. . . ." * We all tend to do queer things in extraordinary situations; it is queerness in ordinary situations which makes for what we call abnormality. True normality, psychologically speaking, is very close to mediocrity. It presents a picture of almost automatic life—every one doing things in the same way. It is a matter of congratulation (to quote Jastrow, again) that we are not all "hopelessly sane—irrevocably bound to routine responsiveness, immune to all inspiration, fated to a bare, regular, simple treadmill routine of conduct." If we were so bound we should have no artists, no poets, no writers, no musicians, no students even, and certainly no saints. Rather than to lose all these we can easily afford to risk a few sinners.

Among the desirable expressions of abnormality, we must place the tendency to "carry on," a persistency of attitude in thought and

* Joseph Jastrow: *Character and Temperament.* But to the above Dr. Jastrow adds, "or at the more critical periods of development or stress." I have quoted the passage only so far as it serves my idea.

action which brings results in spite of obstacles; a tendency very different from that so common to many of us and so deadening to progress, by virtue of which we tend to avoid all unpleasant effort. Again, the nervous man is the trouble-finder of this world, as well as the trouble-taker, and he thus becomes the forerunner, if not the actual elaborator, of improvement.*

And now the other side! Of course we can have nothing in this world without paying for it—these heightened sensibilities and disproportionate reactions may end in catastrophe, and this "carrying on" may result in exhaustion. The nervous man walks a very narrow path, and it is almost a "toss up" whether it shall lead him to success and to honour, or whether he shall fall into the mire of illness, or disgrace.

Neurasthenia and Hysteria

Neurasthenia, or nerve exhaustion, in its simplest form, is a fatigue superinduced by worry. It is the fatigue of a nervous man, a worrying man, one who has carried on to excess. Work without worry leads only to a fatigue which can be recovered from by the simple process of

* Wilfred Lay, *op. cit.*

rest. But why qualify the statement? All fatigue can be recovered from by rest—the trouble with the worrying man is that he can not get that rest. When a worrying man with sensitive nerves, or, maybe, with a deficient nerve force, works beyond his safe limit, the result is an ill man, an exhausted man, a man with nerve exhaustion. Furthermore, as the nerves determine nearly everything else in the body, this man with the nerve exhaustion will have a lot of other things too—quickly fatigued muscles and mind, a poor digestion, heart troubles, headaches and backaches, and so on, beyond computation. Worry and dyspepsia are two cute little beings which nearly always trip-it along hand in hand.

In the more pronounced cases of neurasthenia, those which drag on for months and years despite physical rest and good hygiene and removal of all evident worries, we must look for other causal factors. These may be found in glandular and other organic defects, or in toxic states—poisoning of the system from local foci of infection, the teeth, the tonsils, or hidden abscesses. Or, and of this only shall I speak, the trouble may be in the subconscious mind of the victim, in the existence there of mental conflicts which by their presence prevent that harmonious mental action which good health demands.

Where are these conflicts—in what do they consist? I have spoken of our storing away in the unconscious things we had no immediate use for, but intend to use some day—we put there other things, too, things we do not want at all, which we would be glad to be rid of, and which we truly hope never to see again. For instance, a certain experience comes to us; it is a shocking experience; we can not fit it in with our other experiences; and so we bury it—shove it down deep into the unconscious. At least we try so to do, and we may succeed, we may forget it; or, we may leave it just below the surface where it remains only partially covered. But whether deeply buried or only partially buried, this shocking experience, be it noted, still retains, like all the rest of the unconscious, its power of influencing the conscious mind. Our conscious effort may get it out of our conscious life, but it will remain in the unconscious, a source of irritation and of contradiction, and of interference with the harmonious workings of the mind—a source, in short, of conflict. In the majority of cases of neurasthenia it is with the conscious or semiconscious worry that we are concerned, the worry in the background of our thoughts, which keeps nagging away until we are fairly distracted—the deeper conflicts, the truly unconscious worries, if we may use such an expression, tend to other disorders. No harmonious action of mind can be possible with these unsolved problems always in troublesome evidence. Every action and every thought becomes fatiguing; will and effort are required to effect them—no wonder the man breaks and becomes ill! It is the consciousness of an act that fatigues, while automatism makes for rest. Become deliberately conscious of any movement and the muscles soon tire. When a novice in public has occasion to walk before an audience, his walking becomes conscious and difficult—so here, in neurasthenia, all action quickly leads to exhaustion.

There are opposing schools of thought in medical practice—to one the buried conflict is everything, to the other the organic basic alone is important. But why try to force all cases into one class? Nature and science do not readily lend themselves to arbitrary classifications, though, unfortunately, quasi-scientists do! The fact, as we have it in neurasthenia, is the existence of the exhausted nerves—a state of exhaustion which can not obtain that rest which good health requires. Whether this condition be due to an inherent nerve weakness, to an organic irritation, to a glandular disturbance, or to a toxemia, or whether it be due to an unsolved mental problem, it will be the duty of the wise physician to determine.

In *hysteria* we again meet the buried complex, and here the advocates of this theory are especially at home. The conflicting problem, in hysteria, is conceived to be deeply buried, meaning by this, literally, that it is something so foreign to our other experiences that we simply can not tolerate it at all, and so we inhibit it, shut it off, with all of our power, from reaching consciousness. Or, the problem is due to some innate hidden tendency which has not been properly oriented with our conscious life and, for this reason, has been prevented from expression. The buried complex, however, continues its influence and does make itself manifest, but, in hysteria, only after having undergone change into some form less antagonistic to our conscious life. The force of the impulse must find expression; it can not do so in its original form, so it becomes converted into a new and, to the personality of the individual, a more acceptable form. Unpleasant enough this new form may be, but it is at least a possible form, not impossible as was the original.

The Freudians claim that the buried complex, or impulse, is always one of sex. Others, who have only partly accepted Freud's teachings, find that *any* ordinary, natural, primitive impulse, if sufficiently foreign to our conscious intention, may be equally a source of conflict— the fear complex, for example, which was so frequently the cause of hysterical breakdowns during the war.

Let us consider one form of "shell-shock," as a first example of what we mean by hysteria. Two men go to the Front. They have had several months of hard training under conditions foreign to all previous experience, and, we will say, foreign to their desires. From the moment of their induction into the service they have been under nerve strain; they are non-militant by nature, and have no real disposition for war; the position they find themselves in is due solely to patriotism, or to the draft. Deep, in their souls lies buried primitive fear—not fear of death, maybe, so much as fear of the unknown, and fear of not doing their duty. This strong, natural, instinctive sense, by which we guard our persons and our pride, is not a shameful thing—it is common to all who are neither fools nor philosophers. But, filled as our two men are with this subconscious dread, what do we see? We see them laughing and joking, and apparently indifferent to death, ready in a flash for a trip ''over the top,'' or for any dangerous duty which offers. Imagine the conflict going on here—the powerful instinct of self-preservation facing the unceasing menace which surrounds! And think of the laugh and the brave readiness of the external reaction; and think, too, of the wet, and the cold, and of the deadly fatigue, and of the death which surrounds them; and last, but not least, of the seemingly hopeless, unending continuance before them.

Then comes a day when our two men are caught in an explosion. They are buried in a mass of trench débris. They are dug out by their comrades. Up to this moment the two have had the same feelings, and have reacted in equally proud manner to the necessities of their life, but now—Private A. is found to have a crushed knee; Private B. is sound and whole. Private A. is placed upon a stretcher and, smiling and joking, is carried back to the rear. No wonder he is happy! What is a little physical pain? His problem is solved! He has fought his fight, and he is through!

But what of Private B.? He sees his companion go—and he is left. He must again take up his rifle, and "carry on" as before. For him there is no relief, and he is tired beyond words—his very soul is both tired and sick. He is nervous, and ragged, and shocked. Suddenly something breaks within him. What is this? He finds that he can not move one of his feet— he is paralyzed! The thought comes to his mind with a pleasant rush—and now he, too, goes back to the hospital, a "shell-shock" case. His subconscious mind has won, and his problem has been solved in its favour. There is no nerve injury; there is no organic cause for the paralysis, he has hysterical paralysis; but, so far as he is concerned, it is real, for he can not now move his foot. I say his subconscious has won. It has obtained for him that which he truly desired, but which he would not, in his conscious mind agree to, nor acknowledge. This is hysteria.

Note the difference, here, between hysteria and neurasthenia. In the latter the conscious mind retains a control, albeit a sickly one, and life goes on in a forced, difficult progress, a process of continuous struggle. In hysteria, on the other hand, it is the subconscious complex which wins in the conflict, and, which, breaking through into the conscious, in some modified form, there attains its desire.

In the illustration just given, the victim was prepared for his hysteria by outrageous strain. In civil life such a cause must be rare, and yet hysteria is a common disease. We must look, then, for some other cause, and this we shall generally find in the inherent disposition of the sufferer. Some individuals, from inheritance of nerve weakness and of nerve irritability, or through development of the same by illness, seem to lack the normal degree of conscious control. They exhibit an increased susceptibility to suggestion, and respond in an exaggerated manner to all mental impressions. Their nerves are sensitive, and their excitability great, but their control is deficient. This is the hysterical tendency—few families are lacking in examples. This is the hysterical tendency, but it is not hysteria. To develop the latter, the buried complex and its conflict seem necessary. It is the buried complex, the hidden unconscious wish, which, breaking through into consciousness makes itself manifest in some one of its protean disguises. Here, now, we find, as in shell-shock, all those remarkable exhibitions, generally in the physical field, such as pains, contractures, spasmodic movements, faintings, fits, paralyses, and even blindness and deafness.

The hysteric patient has a pretty tough time of it in this life—and so does the family! The symptoms are often so unreasonable, so perverse, and so unnecessary, and, moreover, so opportune for the patient, that the latter is constantly under suspicion. The term hysterical becomes, unjustly, a reproach; it would seem as though the patient *must* be pretending, as though he surely could be well, if only he would. Let us take an example from everyday life. The household is confronted with the spring cleaning—but the hysteric daughter develops a sick headache, and has to be waited on herself, while the others do all the work. Now this is enough to make any one mad! The others, the healthy members of the household, feel that the headache is a pretence, that it is assumed to avoid the unpleasant labour. Well, they are right, in a way, it is assumed—it would not have come on had there been a matter of pleasure in prospect—but it is, nevertheless, beyond the power of the patient to prevent its coming on, and it is real and distressing now that it is here. In other words, the headache is a response to an impulse from the subconscious mind (in this case, a desire to avoid work) but the conscious mind will not acknowledge this. The patient says, and actually feels, in her conscious thought, that she would be glad enough to do the work if only she could; but her unconscious desire is stronger than her conscious, and, being antagonistic to this, accomplishes its end in a roundabout way—the headache is the result. The unconscious wins. The wish which could not be admitted into consciousness attains its end by a disturbance of the physical health.

As has been said, this is outside of the patient's power of control; she has not the mastery of her subconscious desire. The distaste for work may have been, and probably was, just as strong in the subconscious minds of the others, but this they were able to successfully over-rule. The patient with hysteria can not so over-rule; her conscious mind condemns the wish, but her unconscious mind avoids this condemnation by a process of displacement, or "conversion," and attains its end in a roundabout way. All this doubtless sounds bizarre and surprising enough when first considered, but the hypothesis has stood the test of much investigation, and has, moreover, led to a method of cure, to be referred to shortly.

.   .   .   .

I have given only simple manifestations of hysteria, and, in fact, prefer to limit the term to cases of this type. There are, however, many allied diseases which for the sake of some completeness should be mentioned here. All of these, together with hysteria and neurasthenia, may be classed as "psychoneuroses." We have here the so-called psychasthenias, where some one subconscious impulse of persistent nature *habitually* breaks through the weakened conscious control, and gives rise to what are known as "obsessions" and "compulsions." Thus, the patient may have a compelling desire to steal (kleptomania), or a desire to set fire to things (pyromania); or an obsession of indecision (*folie de doute*), where he struggles helplessly between alternately presenting possible courses of action. In this last affliction, for instance, the patient may spend an hour choosing which suit he shall wear; or as long, even, in deciding which shoe he shall put on first. He is never sure that he has properly turned off the gas, and he will try a locked door a dozen times to make sure that it really is locked.

Again, a fear-habit may be established in some particular direction, as, for example—a fear of being in a closed place (claustrophobia). a fear of open places (agoraphobia), a fear of dirt (mysophobia), a fear of fire (pyrophobia), a fear of the dark (nyctophobia), a fear of thunder storms (astraphobia), or a fear of death (thanatophobia). Allied to these is hatred of intellectual effort (misologia), which would, however, like oniomania (a desire to spend money), seem to be perfectly normal with youth.

In that very unpleasant disease known as the "anxiety neurosis" there is an unreasonable, unfounded sense of impending calamity, with all the physical manifestations and mental sufferings of fear, indefinable, vague, and unknowable. Anxiety is, moreover, a symptom of many of the other disturbances, and in many cases is directly traceable to organic errors, especially to over-activity of the thyroid gland.

Somnambulism, or better, as the French call it, *automatisme ambulatoire*, with partial or complete loss of memory (amnesia) is comparable with the hypnotic states. There may be, too, a "splitting of the personality" where one group of ideas and their associations becomes dominant, and the patient lives for a time entirely within this group, all others being then quiescent and, therefore, forgotten. Passing from life within this limited group, back to the normal life of the mind as a whole, and *vice versa,* gives us the cases of so-called dual personality.

Finally, we may mention here, though of a different class, the "psychopaths"—the moral degenerates, sexual monsters, and "pathological liars"—partially cases of bad inheritance, and partially cases of profound mistraining. In some of these there is a deficient mentality, with an inability to build up sentiments; in others the mentality is fair, or excellent, and sentiments are formed, but they are bad ones. Normal desirable tendencies may be lacking, or, more characteristically, perverted. But, whatever the cause, the result is an antisocial being not guided by those standards upon which the rest of mankind lean for support.

We are merely suggesting some of the complexities of our subject in mentioning these classes of the abnormal—their full discussion belongs to medical psychology; and, even there, there will be found but little agreement between authors. Those who desire only well-defined knowledge had best steer clear of this subject altogether. Probably the best opinion of the day is that which places the *origin* of the psychoneuroses in the organic disturbances of the body, and their *development* in the patient's peculiarities of mind. Two factors seem to be necessary for the production of the average case—the mental, and the physical—but, if we regard mind as dependent upon the physical condition of the brain and nerves, then even this distinction becomes rather vague.

In closing this section let us remark, to quiet certain thoughts that may have arisen with some of my readers, that but few of us have not experienced something of the symptoms described. These symptoms are not in themselves evidence of an abnormal mind, they come to us all, especially in times of fatigue, and in illness—it is only when they have become inordinately persistent and uncontrollable that we reach the abnormal.

Freud

It was mentioned under hysteria that the theory of the hidden complex with the resulting mental conflict had led to a method of cure. The reference was to the Freudian psychanalysis. In a sentence the principle is this—if the mental disease is the product of a hidden, conflicting, and irritating complex, unearth and unravel the latter, and the disease will be gone. Psychanalysis is thus an attempt to bring back to full consciousness the buried problem, to bring it back, to expose it to light, to explain it, to examine it philosophically, and, as a result, to rob it of its importance. The idea is fascinating and promising, for, as a matter of fact, many of these buried experiences date from early life, and it is often only necessary to discover them to find that they are, in themselves, perfectly harmless. A child may have an experience, it may be entirely misunderstood, and may be, to the child, very shocking. It may have been given a strong emotional value by the child, and it may retain this value until unearthed years later, when, on examination, its actual trivial nature is revealed.

Parents are sometimes responsible for this state of affairs—a child may have some insignificant sexual experience, an exposure of the person, for instance.* It really means nothing to the child, and calls for only kind advice from the mother; but suppose that the mother expresses horror and shame for the child, punishes her, and forbids her, in awe-compelling manner, ever to do such a shameful thing again; forbids her even ever to mention it—the whole question is now on a wrong basis. The innocent childlike action receives in the child's mind an unhealthy accentuation, and yet must be repressed! For weeks, long after the parent has

* Cf. Wilfred Lay, *op. cit.*

226

forgotten the incident, the child continues to brood over her sin, and then finally buries it in her subconscious mind, all wrapped up in its revolting winding sheet. Here is the laying of a buried complex which may, however, unfortunately, be heard from again. Suppose now this experience be later unearthed—in the better judgment of more mature years it is recognized for what it was truly worth, namely, nothing; or, if still painful, it may be that, with our larger experience of life, we can now do what we could in nowise do before, fit it in, treat it rationally, and regard it with disarming understanding.

Psychanalysis has brought relief to many; it has often swept away unreasonable fears, and, honestly and skilfully used, it has often provided a better philosophy of life—but, unfortunately, it has elements of danger. It is so extremely personal, and involves so much of sex, that it may do great harm through suggestion; and, moreover, it calls for a degree of intimacy between patient and physician which is in itself a menace, especially as the patient is generally of a neurotic and suggestible type. Again, it is not, and can not be, universally applicable. Aside from the possible, underlying organic basis for the nervous affection, the fact, just mentioned, that the patient is often inherently and mentally abnormal, renders the conflict but an incident of the disease, and not at all its sole cause. One who is by inheritance, or otherwise, temperamentally and organically wrong can not be cured by the removal of any one disturbing element.

The keynote of Freudianism is sex, and this I have not felt it necessary to dwell upon. But let us consider for a moment the nature of Freud's position.

Much of what I have ascribed to the subconscious, or unconscious, using these terms indifferently, is placed by the Freudians in what they call the "foreconscious" mind. For them the "Unconscious" is the deepest substratum of all, and consists, if we may use such loose language, of *desire*, sexual desire. This is the "libido," the urge of sex, the urge of life, the instinctive wish aimed at propagation. The expression of this wish society has tabooed, and it has, therefore, been shoved back, or down, into the unconscious, whence it can again emerge only after transformation into some more acceptable form. From the powerful urge of this wish, and its efforts toward expression, with its suppressions, and repressions, and transformations, the followers of Freud have

228

built up a system of psychology. From the psychopathies, psychasthenias, neurasthenias, and hysterias, to dreams, everyday errors, blunders of speech, and forgettings, all are traceable to this unconscious sex urge.

Now, to its devotees, this system of Freud seems all satisfying, and here is where, as it seems to the writer, the error lies. As a system it is complete only if we focus our attention on just these particular manifestations mentioned above, and leave out altogether the major part of the phenomena of mind. The fallacy in the Freudian idea lies in its pretension to be all explanatory and all embracing. That the sex impulse is explanatory of much, few will deny; but that it is explanatory of all, few will agree. As a consequence, the Freudian school, though prominent, is a small one—consisting of a small body of earnest students who are being carried away by the enthusiasm which attends all discovery, and who are pushing on to an extreme whither the rest of us can not be persuaded to follow.

Naturally much that we find in the unconscious mind, being elemental in character, has that startling quality which we commonly call brutal. If sex there looms largely, it is no wonder, as the sexual is probably the strongest of all of our inherited instincts. It is not, then, be it observed, because Freud is sexual and shocking that we object to him; science can not be advanced, nor approached even, if we are to recoil from a truth because it is unpleasant. There is no uncleanness in any honest scientific inquiry, no matter what the subject may be.

From the theoretical standpoint it is easy to conceive of sex attraction as the ultimate basis of all material animal life, as it is, we know, the means of life's continuance. But this is, to me, not a useful concept of life—and the value of any concept must be determined by its use to us. Life has long outgrown the purely sexual idea. It has become vast and complex, and must be recognized and studied in all of its complexity. One can not hope to understand life, as it actually exists, by the consideration of but one factor, even though this one factor be both old and important. In the discussion of the sexual instinct, earlier in this book, Bergson was referred to—let us follow him, and call the great life urge the *élan vital,* and then let us regard sexual desire as but one manifestation of this great force. Again, however, on the other hand, do not let us be afraid to face actual sex problems when they arise. Many, very many, go through life with but vague and erroneous notions on the subject, and oftentimes to their sad detriment. In these cases psychanalysis has sometimes led to helpful readjustments, and to a healthier understanding of life in general.

I have given only Freud's theory of the conflict, and of the unconscious mind. It may be of interest, in closing, to refer to some derivations from his original idea. To Freud, as we have found, the unconscious is made up of sexual desire, largely infantile or primitive, and the conflict is between this hidden desire and the conscious mind. To Adler, the conflict is between the unconscious *ego* and the oppressions of an artificial consciousness. To Jung, the unconscious is made up largely of the inherited fancies of the race, and includes both repressed elements and those which have never yet become conscious. The conflict, here, is between the adapted socialized functions of the conscious mind, and the, as yet, unsocialized, undifferentiated co-functions of the unconscious inheritances. To express it more simply, it is a conflict between that part of us which has become civilized, and that part of us which remains in the primitive state. If we can imagine a man of the Pleistocene Age suddenly brought into contact with the present, we know how difficult would be his adjustment to the modern conditions. Such a Pleistocene man we have, each of us, within us. In one who tends toward thoughtful introspection, one whom we call an introvert, the struggle is between the conscious thought and the unconscious feeling; while in one who tends toward action, the extrovert, it is between the conscious feeling and the unconscious thought. Jung's conception is in agreement with much of the position taken throughout this book, though his sexual interpretations are decidedly at variance with it.

Insanity

Viewed psychologically, insanity may be defined as a mental disease developing such marked and persistent departures from the normal that the whole personality of the individual has become altered. Krafft-Ebing, from the anatomical standpoint, defined it as a diffuse disease of the brain, accompanied with nutritive changes, and with inflammatory and degenerative processes. However we may choose to define—and definition here is peculiarly difficult—it is evident that we are now dealing with a serious brain affliction; not with that which is simply not sane, not with a functional disease only, but with one deeply seated organically.

As in all other mental disorders, there are generally two elements involved—the predisposing, and the exciting. The predisposing are the inherited and acquired abnormalities of the individual, while the exciting are to be found in the storms and stresses of life. Of these two, the first must positively be present, but, not always being evident, it is often overlooked, and it is the second, the exciting cause, itself relatively unimportant, that is in popular belief generally alone held responsible. Thus we hear of persons "going insane" from grief and from disappointment, from fear and from shock; but, while it is true that without something of these the disease might never have developed, it is equally true that none of them alone can bring it on. Storm and stress factors enter into the development of practically all mental disorders, both mild and severe, but they are only *factors*, the ultimate causes lie deeper.

We can not, then, diagnose insanity from the exciting cause—nor are the symptoms characteristic; neither by symptoms nor by symptoms plus the apparent cause, can insanity be differentiated from other mental disturbances. For our differentiation we are driven back to

233

the underlying first cause, the brain's organic predisposition, and it is upon this we must concentrate our attention—upon this, and upon the *course* of the disease. The predisposing organic factor can not, indeed, be always discovered, and its demonstration and proof is still more often lacking; but that it is always there the writer firmly believes. With the inheritance of diseased germ cells from the mother or father, or as the result of some devastating acquired disease of the patient, the brain has either been rendered abnormal in development, or has later undergone some permanent damage. What happens? With these anomalies of brain growth, with these peculiarities, microscopic, maybe, of structure, we get disturbed, or blocked, associations, and exaggerations and retardations of function. We have periods of inordinate excitement, and periods of depression; we have distorted ideas of personality, and loss of memory, and loss of orientation. There are illusions, misinterpretations of the senses; hallucinations, images formed "without external cause"; and delusions, unreasonable beliefs maintained against all reasonable proof to their contrary.

As prominent among the causes for these abnormal developments, I would place syphilis.

It is not always demonstrable—probably not
more than fifteen per cent of insanity is now
traced to this origin—but syphilis often leaves
scars when the disease itself can no longer be
proven. Syphilis is common, and insanity is
rare; the disease is often expended upon other
organs than the brain, and it does not always
cause the transmission of a diseased germ cell;
but when it does attack the brain, or when it
does cause transmission of diseased germ cells,
some form of profound brain disturbance, generally permanent, is bound to result.

Alcohol has frequently been accused of "filling our insane asylums," but this is only one of
those exaggerated statements so beloved by the
prohibitionists. All enthusiasts tend to this
kind of utterance. Prolonged alcoholism must
naturally incline toward lowered vitality in off-
spring, but it does not give rise to insanity—
unless the delirium of the patient in acute alcoholism be so counted. Neurotic, illy balanced
people have often a physiological call for alco-
holic stimulation, and the use of alcohol is with
them a symptom, not a cause. "Alcoholism is
a sign of something, but by no means necessarily a cause for anything." * It is a sign of

* R. G. MacRobert: *The Journal of the American Medical Association,* April 10, 1920.

our over-civilized life, with its mental fatigues, and of a craving for rest and relaxation, which can be obtained, by many, in this one way only. That it does not truly improve the health is too subtle an objection to appeal to the labouring man; he feels better after its use, and that is enough for him. As a matter of fact, alcohol, in moderation, brings about relaxation in a tired man, and, by this effect, it opens the way to the true physiological rest which his body demands. It has saved many a man from a breakdown, and has saved society many a strike, and other anti-social expression of tired and irritated nerves.

The chief among the insanities may be included under the following four types; paranoia, the manic-depressive group, paresis, and dementia precox—and, there might be added, the familiar dementia of old age. *Paranoia* is marked characteristically by delusions; first of hypochondriac and depressive nature, and then of suspicion and of persecution, and, ultimately, of inordinate self-importance. The last stage, that of importance, the stage of the exaggerated ego, is a natural successor to the second, that of persecution, for one is not persecuted unless one be important—the deduction is both logical and reasonable. The whole has been summed up tersely, as: *"Il fuit; il se defend; il attaque."* The *manic-depressive group*, including, in its typical form, the "cyclic" insanities, shows alternating periods of melancholia and of mania, of depression and of excitement, with, often, intervals of normal life. *Paresis*, a gross syphilitic disease, begins generally with loss of application, with loss of judgment, and with a general nervous irritability, and passes, in the typical case, to a second stage, known as the expansive, or grandiose. It is here we meet with the Queen Victorias and Emperor Napoleons of the madhouse, with the possessors of fabulous wealth, and of miraculous power. The final stage in paresis is one of dementia and stupidity. *Dementia precox*, precocious dementia, is an insanity of puberty and of the young adult. There is here an early breaking down of the mentality; a child, after several years of normal existence, gradually becomes nervous, moody, irritable, inefficient, and shallow; and then, ultimately, silly and stupid.

It is evident, as has already been said, that there are no symptoms which are in themselves characteristic of insanity. The course of the disease is, however, always suggestive, for the end is, in nearly all cases, no matter what the beginning, a profound dementia, a more or less complete loss of mental power, together with other, physical, signs of degeneration.

Not all inmates of asylums are insane, in the narrow sense which I have adopted. Many of the more serious functional disturbances tend to become permanently fixed, and may so incapacitate the victim that confinement, or as we might better call it, protection, in an institution becomes desirable. Unfortunately there is a stigma attached to the suspicion of mental disease. Were it not so, were it regarded as are other diseases, relief from early symptoms would be more often sought, and doubtless many would thereby be spared the final collapse. Clinics for the early relief of mental disorders are now being established in our larger cities, and to them the heartiest encouragement should be given. Patients of wealth have always been able to secure proper refuge in private sanatoriums, but these institutions are necessarily closed to those of lesser means. The public asylums, generally speaking, are good—some of them better than many of the private—but to obtain entrance thereto a commitment by court is required. The patient who is mentally ill can not obtain the aid he so much needs without being first stigmatized publicly as an abnormal being. In fact, he must be

labelled as *insane,* for nothing short of this will
satisfy the law. No wonder such aid is accepted
as a last resort only—when it is too late, when
the disease itself has become fixed and hopeless.

. . . .

It is a common remark, born, I believe, of
our envy, that genius and insanity are closely
related. The Emperor Charles V. had
"epilepsy," so did Peter the Great. Cæsar
had hysterical convulsions, so had Napoleon.
Pascal suffered from many nervous disabilities,
and Richelieu was a victim of periodic melancholia. Mozart had fainting fits, and died, at
thirty-six, of a disease of the brain. Chopin
and Beethoven were decidedly "queer." Swift,
Johnson, Cowper, Southey, Coleridge, Byron,
Lamb, DeQuincey, and Poe are some of
the many men of letters who have suffered
from abnormality. But what does this sig-
nify? These men, and many other of our
great ones, are not like the rest of us—
that is why they are great. They have
quick sympathies, great imaginations, fine
keenness of perception, and very ready associations—their minds are, in short, super-minds
—but for this they must pay. The question
has been already discussed, or at least referred

to, in our opening remarks on the abnormal. There is a vast difference between genius and insanity; the two are antipodal—nor do I refer now to the organic cause for the latter. They both do, indeed, depart from the normal, and both exhibit great activity of mind; but the genius has a wealth of images to draw upon, and has control of these images, and can weave them into thousands of patterns. The insane, on the other hand, are marked by paucity of material; with them the same patterns tend to recur indefinitely. Only in the first stages of an insanity coming on in an educated person, might there be any confusion. It would be difficult to say, for example, at least from his writings, just when Dean Swift gave the first signs of his mental disease. Here, in a case like this, a mind richly stored, when stimulated by disease, may rise temporarily to higher flights of fancy, as well as to increased productive activity. But the added power is soon lost; the mind begins to shut in on itself, to lose control of associations, and, finally, to lose the associations themselves. All but a few of the brain patterns become destroyed, and the control of these few soon passes out of the power of their possessor.

The resemblance between genius and in-

sanity, psychologically speaking, is merely that both are departures from the normal average of reaction—they are in no other way similar.

CHAPTER XII

THE CROWD

GUSTAVE LEBON characterized "the coming era," that very evidently now here, as the Era of Crowds; while I, in my opening remarks have styled it one of Militant Minorities. Our thoughts really "jump together"; there is no contradiction here; we have merely concentrated on two different features of the same phenomenon. The minority and the crowd are intimately correlated in action; the crowd is helpless until led, and the minority is powerless without the crowd which it engages to perform its will. Witness Russia today with its very small group of militant "red" despots, and its servile, helpless, red-following masses.

But what is a crowd? Well, psychologically, it is a very different thing from that which the word ordinarily recalls to mind. In the ordinary sense it is a "confused multitude" (Stormonth), a mass of humanity, generally conceived to be upon its feet, and moving—a mob —a word which itself expresses motion, being but the apocope of *mobile,* and a slangy abbreviation of *mobile vulgus*. Psychologically, however, while the familiar mob is included, the term crowd is enlarged to embrace all groups of individuals who, by the act of grouping, have resigned a something of their individual character, and have obtained, not new attributes, but a new type of behaviour, a new, or rather very old, manner of reaction. We are begging the question is a statement such as this, but its development will follow.

In this psychological interpretation of the term we must place with crowds all groups that have become conscious of their existence as such, whether they be formed for a purpose or by chance. Conclaves, parliaments, congresses, holiday seashore crowds, and lynching parties will all be found to have something in common, and it is this something which makes the crowd, psychologically speaking. More than this, under certain conditions actual contact, even, is not necessary; and a nation or any widely scattered group may still be swayed by the rules of the mob. The fervid inauguration of the Crusades in Europe offers an historical example of this.

In all crowds there are, of course, limiting differences, special and particular determinants of action, certain likely types of behaviour, and yet—and this is why the various kinds may all be placed together—there is also a certain resemblance. All of these groups, heterogeneous or homogeneous, formed for a purpose or by accident, tend to a type of reaction which points to that something they all hold in common. It is this mental unity, this mass-mind, which we must try to discover.

The men of a group, and it does not have to be a large group (two is company, three is a crowd, would about express it), by their union form a compound, much as the chemical elements unite to form their compounds.* The mind of a crowd is in no sense equal to the sum of the minds of its members, nor even to an average of the same; it is, instead, on a plane distinctly below that average. A new compound has been formed in the union, but this new compound lacks much of the value of its component parts. Is this doubted? Note the insane violence of an angry mob, the cowardly brutality of a lynching party, and the stupidity of many legislative acts. Who of us has not applauded some vacuous platitude of a public speaker, and then wondered with shame, after returning home,

* LeBon: *The Crowd, A Study of the Popular Mind.* London. It was not by chance that this chapter opened with the name of Gustave LeBon. The name of this distinguished French ethnologist and psychologist will always be associated with the psychology of the crowd. He has left little for us to add.

THE CROWD

what it was that impelled our silly enthusiasm? The angry mob may be made up of peace-loving shopkeepers, and the cause of their anger may be, personally, of no interest to them whatsoever. The lynching party may be composed of some of the "gentlemen" of the community, or at least of men who ordinarily and individually talk a lot about their honour and courage. The legislators may be level-headed men of capability who individually recognize their legislative act as absurd.

The mind of the crowd is not only inferior, it often possesses no reason at all. It is primarily emotional;* it is swayed by trivialities; it is intolerant of criticism; impatient, suggestible, and credulous. It lynches a man on the most paltry evidence; it passes laws which it hopes will not be put into effect; it awards praise and blame without awaiting the facts; and it thinks, if it thinks at all, only after all is over. When the Greek assembly ordered the massacre of the citizens of Mytilene it acted against reason and contrary to its own interests. Then came night and a recovery, for some, of their social sense and humanity, with

* I have referred to the word *mob* as being derived from *mobile*—note that *emotion* too, is expressive of movement. There is exhibited here the usual deep psychological intuition which lies behind so much of our language.

245

the result that the following day the crowd is led to revoke its inhuman decree—which it does with the same enthusiasm it had exhibited in originally passing it. When the assembly, acting on like impulse, after the battle of Arginusae, ordered the deaths of its victorious generals, because of their rumoured neglect to care for the bodies of the dead, the sentence was unfortunately executed before the reaction to sanity was obtained. It was the mob that without reason demanded that Christ rather than Barabbas should die. It was mob psychology that committed the September massacre (in 1792), and which then sought reward for its "patriotic act." It is the psyche of the mob which causes a crowd to yell itself hoarse over the victory of some politician whom they do not know and whose policies and intentions must ever remain beyond their powers of appreciation. It is the same psyche which leads to the hue and cry, to the careless destruction of property by holiday mobs, and to the cruelty of revolutionary tribunals.

It is mob psychology which explains the explosive laugh in the theatre when the actor, or, better still, the actress, exclaims "Hell!" or "Damn!" It is as though an electric button were touched, so quick is the response, and so regular. As a matter of fact it is receptive primitive sensibility that is so touched off. The audience is *ready* to react, it is *ready* for the emotional response, and these primitive exclamations offer just the kind of stimulus needed.

So with lynching, it is mob psychology, or, in other words, as it is here exhibited, a primitive blood lust, that explains the conversion of a group of presumably respectable citizens into a cowardly gang of ruffians. Lynching is not, as is so commonly believed, an outburst of righteous indignation. It too often follows some trivial offence, and is by no means always a punishment for heinous crime.

It is, in part at least, mob psychology which explains how a nation can pass an Eighteenth Amendment, and then set its wits to work to evade it. It is the mob which burns men as sorcerers, and which cries for the blood of unsuccessful patriots, and which then erects monuments to their memory. It is, too, the mob which proclaims men as heroes and then subjects them to cavilling criticism. While one member of the committee pins a medal on the hero's breast, another pins, on the tail of his coat, a placard inscribed, "Please Kick Me"— or, at least, so once said "Mr. Dooley." The ceremony over, as the victim retires, the placard alone is to be seen, and the crowd joyously accepts its invitation.

To understand the psychology behind these facts we must recall the complexity of man's nature, the vast inheritance of primitive tendencies, and the variety of his possibilities of expression. We know that the forest-past is but slightly veneered over by the social present, and we know how eagerly man reverts to the easy old patterns. This has been discussed earlier in this book, in the section on Play.

Now, the fact is, when a man becomes part of a crowd he descends several rungs on the ladder of civilization. "Isolated he may be a cultivated individual; in a crowd he is a barbarian —that is, a creature acting by instinct. He possesses the spontaneity, the violence, the ferocity, and also the enthusiasm and heroism of primitive beings, whom he further tends to resemble by the facility with which he allows himself to be impressed by words and images." *
The same thought is expressed, with his accustomed elegance, by Joseph Jastrow: "The collective mental responsiveness proceeds upon the elemental, communal traits of human nature; it reflects the indispensable, the more

* LeBon.

248

THE CROWD

nearly original in mental evolution.'' Indeed,
as he adds, in a measure the primitive psychology of man might be reconstructed from a study
of man's collective actions.

Man, then, does not *take on* anything by becoming a member of a mob; he really *drops*
something, and this something is, socially, his
best part. He becomes simplified by a stripping away of his late accumulations of reason,
and he is carried back to something near his
original state. He thus, moreover, becomes
more positive and direct, and even more under-
standable for those who will read. His actions
now are unhampered by social inhibitions and
he has nothing to fear. But, as has been said,
these are not new attributes that he has gained,
they are merely old ones that have now been
freed. A vari-coloured mosaic may present no
distinct colour impression to the eye, but take
away all colours but one, and that one will be
evident enough. So man in a crowd attains to
the mob psychology and becomes primitive and
emotional, and direct, by a stripping away of
his recently acquired mental additions, such as
reason and deliberation. The passions so loos-
ened may appear gross and unnatural but it is
really, by their freedom from nullifying restraint that they come so into prominence. We

learn something of the possibilities within us
when we yield to the contagion of the crowd,
and the insight so obtained should make us more
humble.

The explanation of this degradation of
the individual by his incorporation into a
crowd seems to me to be contained in a
remark of Schopenhauer, who, speaking of
association in general, says: ''Intercourse
with others involves a process of levelling
down. The qualities which are present in
one man, and absent in another, can not
come into play when they meet.'' Apply this
to a crowd. Cancel those qualities which
are not held in common—the socially best, the
intellectual and fine—and what is left? A few
primitive reactions only, common instincts and
tendencies, left now uninhibited and ready for
expression—and these give you your crowd psychology. It is the innate only which is shared,
and which by contact, emulation, and sympathy
becomes reinforced. That which is merely
reasonable, not being shared, weakens and dies.
Efficient thought, able judgment, high purpose,
these we know to be uncommon attributes, belonging to the few, not the many; they can not
be common in a crowd. All that the members
of a crowd have in common are the original

emotional tendencies with which we all began life.

Such, in my belief, is the essence of crowd psychology, though, of course, it is not all. But it is this which is the characteristic of crowds in general, and the underlying cause of all else that we find. For the rest we are thrown back to a study of the primitive tendencies and to the modifications of these in their collective expression. All emotions enter into prominent play, but certain of them find in the crowd their most appropriate field of activity. Imitation, sympathy, and the gregarious instinct, these three closely related dispositions, are especially active, and from them alone one can explain much of what is observed. Vanity too plays a large part, as is shown by the methods necessary to crowd control, and, also, by the love of the crowd for unrestricted exaggeration. Out of many we have made one, but that one is strong, very strong, for in union there is strength; individual responsibility is lessened or altogether removed, as is, also, the fear of punishment. Each individual becomes both strong and daring; he shares in the strength of the unit of which he has become a part, and he divides his responsibility by the number present. In this he does show, maybe, a glimmer of reason, but it is emotionally arrived at, not a product of conscious thought. Emotion rules all; arguments become futile and empty and tiresome. Generalized sentiments alone appeal, and a popular slogan, if sufficiently vague to be given by each his own interpretation, will outweigh all the facts in the world.

These are, in general, some of the features of crowds, those common to all, though fortunately not always exhibited in their extreme. When we come to consider the *kinds* of crowds, we find, of course, other factors involved. There are, for instance, the temperamental determinants of race. A crowd of Frenchmen, other things being equal, will hardly react in the same manner as will a crowd of English. The Oriental has his manner of responding to a stimulus; the Occidental has his—and so on. Their traditions provide a mould into which they naturally slip, and to which they adjust their reactions. There is a senatorial courtesy; there is a mass-meeting discourtesy; or, to go far afield, note the handclapping of tennis spectators, the yells and "catcalls" of baseball rooters, and the silence of an enthusiastic golf "gallery."

Is crowd action always bad? No, no more than are the emotions all bad; but it is always dangerous, as are all uncontrolled primitive reactions. Our social life today demands a degree of intellectual command over the emotions, and it is precisely in this that the crowd falls below the normal for the individual.

I am not competent to pass upon German etymologies, but Carlyle relates the German *Schwarmerei* (enthusiasm) with "swarmery," the gathering of men into swarms, and speaks of the prodigies they are in the habit of doing and believing "when thrown into that miraculous condition." "Some big Queen Bee," he says, "is the centre of the swarm; but any commonplace stupidest *bee*, Cleon the Tanner, Beales, John of Leyden, John of Bromwicham [Lenin or Trotzky], any bee whatever, if he can happen, by noise or otherwise, to be chosen for the function, will straightway get fatted and inflated into bulk, which of itself means complete capacity; no difficulty about your Queen Bee; and the swarm once formed, finds itself impelled to action, as with one heart and one mind. Singular, in the case of human swarms, with what perfection of unanimity and quasi-religious conviction, the stupidest absurdities can be received as axioms of Euclid, nay, as articles of faith, which you are not only to believe, unless malignantly insane, but are (if you have any honour or morality) to push into practice, and without delay see *done,* if your soul would live!''

The Queen Bee of the swarm, the successful political leader, is, perforce, a born psychologist, a specialist in mob psychology, though he may never have heard of such a thing. He does not feed his audience reason; he does not present arguments—he does not acknowledge that there are two sides to the question. He asserts with emphasis; he reiterates, and he pounds the table. Opponents are fools and rascals. He plays upon all the primitive emotions—the vanities, the fears, the loves and the hates—until, if he has played well, the audience rises with enthusiasm, with *Schwarmerei,* and acclaims him its political messiah. Failing to gain as much in contributions as it had hoped for, one party *accuses* the other of having received too much. It is not a statement of fact that is made, it is an accusation of criminality, and the sympathetic audience thrills with horror—at what? They do not know, but they act as the candidate knew they would act, and that is what he was after.

Slogans become all powerful. ''He kept us out of war'' elected a president. We used to hear, too, of ''A full dinner pail,'' and, long, long ago, of ''An honest dollar.'' The term

"Yellow Peril" used to be good for at least one shudder; just as, today, the European radical unites his mob by frequent reference to "The White Terror." What is the White Terror? The slogan comes down from 1815, but it is used now to describe the humble bourgeoisie whose machinations are represented as aimed at the glories of radicalism!

In the public assembly it is the same. It is *Schwarmerei* that rules, and it is he who best understands the psychology involved who occupies the position of leader. It is *Schwarmerei* that votes away the people's money, and it is this same, plus mob exaggeration and loss of individual responsibility, that makes popular government the most expensive government of all. Are examples of my assertions needed— read the public press or better, the *Congressional Record*.

It is a great game! The only difficulty is, and this is where its sportiness comes in, once started one can not let go. The mob is as fickle as it is emotional; it is emotional to the extreme, and therefore it is fickle to the extreme. Do not think that you can ever recapture a crowd once it has escaped your grasp. "Eloquence is a bit," says Hugo, "if the bit breaks, the audience runs away and makes on till it has thrown the orator . . . instinctively he pulls the reins but this is a useless expedient,'' it only makes the runaway the madder. It is a great game and its fascination is such that with many it is the game only that counts. With many a leader the material rewards are left to the henchmen. Not all politicians are out for the money.

Has not all this a special bearing for us as advocates of democracy? I believe that it has, and a very important one. Since rule by the people must always mean, actually, rule by the few, it behooves us to see to it that our leaders are chosen with care. And they must be leaders in fact, not as is so often the case, themselves mere followers of the mob. ''There go the people,'' exclaimed one Roman Senator to another, on seeing a crowd surge across the forum, ''We are their leaders—let us follow!'' Such leadership is a mere concentration of the mob psychology into the hands of an executive, and makes for transient success only. Intellectual control, conference, and deliberation must be the reliance of democratic government if this is to become what the ideal calls for. The *best* will of the people must be followed, that which is expressed through its best intelligence, and the mob should be guided to agree.

THE CROWD

Psychology has no quarrel with democracy; we all believe at least in the republican form of government, but psychology recognizes its difficulties. Democracy would be easy only were all men angels—and well educated ones at that.

CHAPTER XIII

WE have spoken of the conflict between the subconscious and the conscious mind—there is another conflict, that between the individual and society. From the social standpoint, man is normal or abnormal according as to whether or not he finds himself able and willing to adapt to the social requirements.

Life is a process of adaptation from the moment of birth to that of death; and growth consists in learning our limitations. Our individual claims meet the claims of other individuals, and adjustments become necessary if all are to go on. So it has always been—Adam and Eve doubtless made many mutual compromises; Cain was unable to adjust to Abel, so removed him. He treated Abel as man today has treated the liquor problem—the problem was too big for him, so he killed it. By friction, and clash, and adjustment, society has been moulded, and what we find today is the result of the conflicts, to the present. "Man is born free; and everywhere he is in chains" is the lament of Rousseau; but what does this mean—is it not simply this, that no man is free to do just what he pleases? The desires of man are as the sands of the seashore, and any one of them, unsatisfied, and brooded over with discontent, may become both a grievance and a gyve.

The great problem has always been to unite men, with their strongly individualistic tendencies, into a group, and there keep them happy. Now this can not be done without willing sacrifice on the part of the individual, and many of the supposed "inalienable rights of man" must give way for the sake of the group. The result is that social man finds himself in the end confronted with far more duties than rights. That he does truly gain by serving society is, of course, demonstrable, but that he would gain more by serving himself, seems far more likely to the many. Nor is belief in rights limited to any one class. Note the demand for untrammelled speech by certain college professors. Failing to recognize the obligations assumed by the acceptance of his position, and believing falsely that all independence of expression is good, the college radical demands that he shall be permitted, if he think well of it, to undermine the very institution which gives him a living. According to Johnson, every man has a right to express his opinion, and every one else has a right to knock him down for doing so. This may or may not be a good rule, but these professors who whine when they are punished for defying the college authority might profitably give it a thought. The social spirit is not a common one—it is particularly rare, for instance, among socialists—we have it, as a rule, only when it does not encroach on some hobby of our own. Certain rights we always reserve and refuse to contribute for the social good, but if all such reserved rights were to be extracted together, the social fabric remaining would be but a sorry remnant indeed!

The fact is, the majority still talk of rights and struggle to assert them, and so long as this is so, social unrest must surely continue. The concept of duty, this unpleasant necessity of civilization, once fully grasped, social problems will become soluble—they will even solve themselves. This the masses do not, *and can not* understand, and, led by youthful idealists, whom they necessarily misinterpret, they grumble. They still do obey society's laws, because they must—or, more truthfully, *if* they must—but it is always a matter of compulsion. They are like children who resent the restrictions which their elders place upon them, but

who accept and obey because they are powerless to do otherwise. This is one group, the
largest—here, indeed, we find the most of mankind—but there is another group, too, among
the unsocial. This other is composed of those
who not only do not accept society's duties with
understanding, but who do not accept them at
all; who are, in fact, actively in opposition to
the same. These are the "Reds," a militant
minority who are as individualistic and unsocial
as was primitive man. Strongly in opposition
to all social restraint, if interested in politics
and of some intelligence, they become an-
archists; if not so interested nor mentally able,
they become our professional criminals. These
are the natural criminals, the irreconcilable
enemies of society—the intransigents of the
underworld of crime.

A word as to the relative degrees of intellectuality here exhibited. In thus ascribing a
higher order of intelligence to the anarchist
than to the criminal, we would seem to be going
contrary to the facts, but I believe not. The
so-often commented upon "smartness" of a
criminal is generally nothing more than an indifference to moral issues. Remove the moral
restraint, and many things become easy. While
on the other hand, the insensate actions of an-

archists, and others of like ilk, are often solely due to an extreme narrowness of mind—a very different thing from stupidity. Within a certain very limited field of thought, they may be really able; readers and writers of books, and energetic speakers. Their judgments are worthless, but they are judgments for all that; what they lack is broadness of understanding, and, above all, the social sense—the conception of obligation to society, a conception involving the social ideal of duty. Fundamentally, the Red and the professional criminal have the same attitude toward society, they both propose to exploit it for their individual gain.

In the broadest sense, social inadequacy, like individual abnormality, includes all disability; it includes all who do not or can not contribute to the welfare of society—the aged, the ill, the crippled, the idiot, the imbecile, and the insane. Of these we need not now speak, their social inadequacy is so evident that society excuses them and demands from them nothing. The delinquents, on the other hand, are socially inadequate individuals upon whom society does make demands—demands which they are unwilling or unable to satisfy. Here are those, just mentioned, who have distinctly anti-social dispositions, who regard society malignantly; and here are those who would be willing enough to obey society's behests if they knew how, or but could!

It is this last class which seems to me to be the most important of all. Here are those pathetic individuals, the high-grade imbeciles and morons, who, unrecognized as such, are expected to meet conditions far beyond their best powers. Here, too, are the most of the delinquents which society itself has produced by false economics, and by class greed—the victims of fate. With the high-grade imbeciles and morons we will include those, too, just a little higher in mental achievement, who still find themselves unable for the social struggle. Together these form the permanent children of the race—they are, physiologically, examples of arrested development; they actually do not possess the mentality necessary to permit of their making the associations and adjustments required. They act on impulse, as do children; they have weak inhibitions, and but too slight control of their primitive emotions. The pronounced cases of mental failure, as has been said, are of no moment, for they are recognized and excused from the social demands; but these others, who are not recognized, who drift through life, bumped this way and that, kicked, even, and struck at, or knocked down and trod upon—all because they will not do what they can not do—these are the tragic ones!

Here we find our tramps and our beggars, our professional prostitutes, and many, very many, of our criminals. The tramp is simply one who can not adjust to the high level of average society. He has tried, maybe, several social planes, before he has finally found that to which he is adapted. Here he may live and even be happy, but let philanthropy, or chance, raise him to where he does not belong, and he will break with the strain. Lifted out of his sphere, he goes to pieces mentally and physically; put him back on the plane which is normal for him, and he once more becomes happy. The wholesale dragnet of the draft swept many of this type into the army, and the result of the demands there made upon them has been to fill the government insane asylums—with men who, let alone, might have gone through life in simple contentment. Other hundreds are serving long terms in prison because they, too, were unable to adjust quickly to military discipline; they are being punished because nature had denied them the power of adjustment!

Power of adjustment is relative. Many accomplish it so long as no very difficult problem presents, but when the problem does become too heavy, something happens—one becomes a neurasthenic, another an hysteric, another a dyspeptic, while another, again, becomes a thief, or a murderer. Environment and education will probably determine whether a man of this class shall go to the doctor, or to the gallows. One girl, a high-grade imbecile, but carefully protected from all the problems of life, will be a débutante belle and immensely popular—her vacuous mind exhibiting itself in pretty childish ways which are strongly appealing to the "protecting sex." Another girl, of the same mental plane of feeble-mindedness, confronting the heavy problems of life, problems touching her very existence, problems of food, clothing, and shelter, simply can not meet them—and gives her body as the easiest way out. This girl reaches the hospital and morgue, just about the time that the lucky one is planning her marriage.

But feeble-mindedness aside, what of the environment of the very poor, with its deadly perverting and stunting effect? Listen to Charles Lamb [the quotation has been adapted]: "The child of the very poor does not prattle. No one has time to dandle it, no one thinks it worth while to coax it, to soothe it, to humour it. If it cries it can only be beaten. It never had a toy. It grew up without the lullaby of nurses. It was a stranger to the hushing caress, the attracting novelty. No one ever told to it a tale of the nursery. It had no young dreams. It was dragged up—to live or to die as it happened. It breaks at once into the iron realities of life; it chaffers; it haggles; it envies; it murmurs. It has come to be a woman before it was a child.''

As an infant which has been the victim of severe bodily illness seldom regains full normal vitality, so one which has suffered severe deprivation in the emotional field seldom attains to a normal adult emotional life.

. . . .

The concept "criminal" is a purely legal one.* It tells nothing of the individual, but only society's opinion of him. A thief may be a man of high ideals in the first stage of some mental disease. He may be *unmoral,* and deficient in a sense of social obligation, and of right and wrong, or he may be feeble-minded. He may have stolen when intoxicated, or he may be a kleptomaniac. He may have strong tender emotion and may have been impelled to steal by the necessities of his wife or child. He may be a man of bad inheritances and bad im-

* Cf. William A. White, *Principles of Mental Hygiene.*

pulses; or he may be a man of good inheritances
and good impulses, but all overlaid by bad education and environment. Whatever he is, however, society labels him a criminal, and society's
laws are concerned only with his crime.

Society as a whole, then, discriminates but
little. The criminologist, on the other hand,
would effect some sort of a classification, generally from cause. They tell us that we have:
Born Criminals, those with inborn tendencies of
a strong anti-social nature; Criminals of Education, those with acquired criminal traits;
Criminals of Occasion, those who under economic stress yield, in one way or another, to
temptation; and, finally, Criminals of Passion,
those with strong or uncontrollable emotions.
As to the feeble-minded, they are to be found in
all of these groups.

What is to be done about it? Here we have a
criminal class, the smallest of all our classes in
society, and more troublesome and more costly
to society than all the others put together.
Well, in one sense, society itself makes the criminal. It is the resistance to the laws of society
which constitutes criminality. Each new law
involves certain additional members of society
in its meshes, for each new law calls for new
adjustments and brings in new temptations.

One nation has free trade; another forbids importation except under restriction and tax. What is a natural right in one country is a crime in the other. "I like a smuggler," says Lamb, "he robs nothing but the revenue, an abstraction I have never greatly cared about." I am not criticizing the law—I believe in import revenue myself—I am merely trying to show that it is the law which makes the criminal. The lawyer would persuade us, at least so it would seem from their attitude, that their law is sacred and moral, and that crime and sin are synonymous—but they are not—they are quite other than that! It is the word *law* which introduces the confusion. We use the same word for the ordinations of God, that we use for the edicts of our legislatures! Many of society's laws are purely arbitrary assumptions of the desirable, and only too often these assumptions are both wrong and immoral. I sat recently through a term of the criminal court down in North Carolina. Nearly every case presented was a violation in some form of the liquor law, and would not have been there had there been freedom of liquor traffic. In this same court I saw four boys sentenced to sixty days each on the chain gang—for what heinous offence? Why, for playing "crap"! The court here committed a sin; the boys had committed only a crime.

The position taken by Hegel is simple and adequate as an explanation of much of our attitude toward crime. Hegel places the will of the individual as secondary and unimportant as compared with the will of society. The measure of right and wrong is to be determined by society alone; what is anti-social is *unrecht.* Society triumphs in the penalty. Punishment is not a chastisement, but a just retribution—not a means, but an end—the solemn affirmation of a violated principle. You can not correct a criminal by killing him, but you must kill him to vindicate the social conception.

As regards capital punishment there is, it seems to me, no other defensible attitude. Capital punishment has never, in the United States at least, acted as a deterrent for the more serious crimes; nor did it in England when it followed, for instance, a theft of a sum in excess of ten pence value. With us there is always the chance of acquittal—a major chance, for, as one jurist has remarked, murder in the United States is the safest of crimes. Nor is capital punishment useful as an example to others. One of our wardens recently conceived the idea of having hardened criminals present at executions of the death penalty in his prison. This, it was supposed, would impress them and cower them, and arouse in them generally the determination to lead better lives. What happened was that the solemn silence was broken by hoots and catcalls, and by cries of "When do we eat?" Dr. Paul Aubry, in France (1888), found that of 177 murderers, 174 had previously witnessed executions. A bit of criminal psychology comes in here—"A gallows standing high in the gaze of all the world has some analogy to a throne," says Hugo. But listen to a more authoritative voice. Henry Fielding, who was a judge as well as a writer, has this to say: "No hero sees death as the alternative which may attend his undertaking with less terror, nor meets it in the field with more imaginary glory [than does the professional criminal]. Pride, which is commonly the uppermost passion in both, is in both treated with equal satisfaction. . . . His procession to Tyburn, and the last moments there, are all triumphant; attended with the compassion of the meek and tender-hearted, and the applause of his fellows." * The execution has now been made fairly private, and its glory has thereby been dimmed, but may wardens be restrained

* *An Inquiry into the Causes of the Late Increase in Robbers.*

270

from further experiments in this direction!

To return to Hegel—that his position is not now endorsed seems to me to be evidence of our illogical processes of thought, and of our willingness to substitute cant for honesty; but it is evidence, also, of a nebulous, growing feeling that our whole attitude toward crime may be wrong.

There are two evident responsibilities, that toward the individual, and that toward society. These can not be entirely reconciled, nor has much effort been made in the past to accomplish this feat. Law has theoretically considered society and has forgotten the individual, while philanthropy has considered the individual and has forgotten society. Law has considered the crime, and forgotten the criminal—while philanthropy has considered the criminal alone. Today, happily, a new criminology is coming into being. Today the ideal is to include the two factors corresponding to the actual responsibilities. The new criminology aims, with the older philanthropists, to consider the criminal, but to this duty it adds the protection of society. It now proposes to try the criminal, instead of the crime.

Practically this ideal calls for the complete

reform of our criminal laws, or rather for a complete change in our attitude toward them. It calls for a stripping away of the law's long accumulated concretions, and a remodelling on a rational basis. When one considers the petrified nature of the present tradition-laden forms, the order seems a large one!

What happens under the system as it actually exists? The prisoner stands in court a mere incident of the trial, a sort of impersonation of the crime of which he is accused. He may be the victim of circumstances over which he has had no control, or he may be feeble-minded; he may be any of a dozen things, but *he* is not on trial—only his crime. He is found guilty, and is sent to prison. New friends now come into his life, those strong friends one makes in adversity, but among them, unfortunately, are many who belong to the class of professionals. If he were not criminally inclined before (and he need not have been to get sentenced) he now certainly acquires criminal ideas; if he were so inclined, his criminality becomes confirmed and its technique improved. He is a *number*, a dog which society has cast out; he becomes bitter, and hard, and anti-social to the core. He broods over revenge; he learns new ways in crime, and he eagerly awaits his discharge that he may try them. He is finally released—but he says *au revoir*, not farewell! He goes out into society, commits some improved form of his old crime, and, if the police are again lucky, comes back for another seclusion at the public's expense.

What are some of psychology's suggestions as regards this situation? As a fundamental suggestion, and as a point of departure for others, it declares that the penalty shall be considered not as a punishment of the prisoner, but as a measure for the protection of society. It holds that society, instead of concentrating on revenge, should rather, like a wise parent, interrogate itself as to the errors it may have committed to have produced this erring child; and then, having protected itself so far as is possible, it should seek to bring about reformation. It suggests that judges and lawyers shall be trained in criminal psychology, in order that the prisoner before them may be to them a human problem; and that they shall try the prisoner, and not simply endeavour to fit his crime into section and paragraph of the criminal code. It suggests that there shall be an extension to adults of the experience of the juvenile courts—that the constricting red tape of formal court procedure shall be largely stripped away, that the children of larger growth, also, shall be handled humanely, and that experts shall be in attendance to aid in interpreting the personality of the prisoner. It suggests that, whenever possible without danger to society, first offenders, and those guilty of crime under stress, shall be set free under court supervision. If wrong has been done to another, that wrong shall be righted so far as it can be. Fines paid to the state may have value as punishment, but restitution to the victim of the crime has the double value that it emphasizes also what is here particularly needed—the sense of social responsibility. It is the state's negligence which has made the crime possible, and the state should see to it that the victim's loss is made good.

Where there is commitment to prison, the sentence should be indeterminate; the avowed enemy of society should be held for life, if need be, as are the less dangerous insane; but discharge should always be possible when the prisoner can be certified to as fit once more for the social experiment. Finally, psychology and humanity both suggest that the prison shall be a reformatory in fact; that the professional criminal shall be separated from the chance offender, but that both shall be given every help

THE DELINQUENT

toward mental and physical health; that they
shall receive good food, have proper exercise,
and instruction, learn useful trades, and be generally guided to higher ideals.

It may be said that many of these principles
are already recognized in our better communities—but how many "better communities," in
this sense, have we in this broad land of ours?
We have chain-gangs in the South—to which, as
we have seen, even boys are sentenced, and that,
too, for so trivial an offence as the playing with
dice. The court with a knowledge of criminal
psychology is a curiosity. The crime is still
tried, not the criminal. Experts are hired par-
tisans of one side or the other. The indeterminate sentence is only occasional. No reparation
is possible for the victim but by personal and
costly suit; and punishment leads to the incul-
cation of anti-social, not social, ideas. Prison
discipline is in the hands of politically ap-
pointed "keepers"—often brutes of less social
promise than the men whom they bully.*

I say nothing of the false attitude toward the
plea of insanity, nor of the dishonest use of this
plea as an evasion; nor of the privileged im-

* See Frank Tannenbaum, in *The Atlantic Monthly*, for April,
1920, on *Prison Cruelty*. But compare, also, the article by "Number 13" in the same magazine for August, 1920. This last is a
rather remarkable exposition of the criminal mind.

munity of the rich; nor of the perversion of the state's prosecuting attorney into a persecuting attorney, concerned only with his own personal "success"; nor of that ancient, and honourable, and ridiculous relic, the jury. There are many, many things in court formulas which have no better reason for being than that they were once useful. All this would take us too far afield, and any lawyer will tell you that I am already out of my province, and talking nonsense. However, I am merely presenting the psychological attitude, and if I am giving it too dogmatically this is but for clearness. A naturalist may give an opinion of a pictured flower, and while this opinion may be resented by the artist, and may even be absurd from the artistic point of view, it may still have a value. I return to the jury—it is not exactly a flower, but it is too important psychologically to be omitted. Here it sits—a perfect example of survival—a habit of proud origin, the function of which has gone, the very expression of which has degenerated, and yet which has retained its sentimental place. The jury, today, is still spoken of as the "bulwark of liberty." Originally a conclave of the village sages, then a defence against the arbitrary ruler, we find it, today, a group of men, the majority almost invariably of subnormal type, be-

fuddled and wondering, to whom the whole
court procedure is directed. The opposing at-
torneys play down to its level, and that side
wins which best understands the working of its
collective subnormal mind.

But, after all, the disposal of the criminal is
only one part of the problem. It is important
because it is a practical and present issue which
we must meet, but there is another, more important, and this is the prevention of crime, or,
we might say, the prevention of the criminal.
As in the treatment of other diseases, it is the
preventive measure alone which makes for improvement. All crime can not be prevented—
no matter what reformative measures be used,
there will still remain a residuum of individuals
whose inherent natures will throw them into
conflict with society. But something can be
done, the criminal class can be greatly reduced
—and in this reduction, it seems to me, lies one
of the first duties of the state. The old philanthropy, as has been hinted, does not get very
far; it relieves the individual, and lets the system alone. The only real good it does is to the
soul of the philanthropist, and he could just as
easily get his good elsewhere. Not only has
philanthropy done little good, it has even done
harm, for in many ways it has tended to per-

petuate the abnormal. It has cared for the individual, has kept him on his feet, has supplied him with crutches, and has helped him to marry and to perpetuate his kind. Nature deals with its unfit in a far simpler way—it eliminates them—but philanthropy says, "No! This man is in God's image! He must be preserved!" So philanthropy preserves him, lets him marry —and society becomes burdened with a vast progeny, all of whom, in their turn, must be cared for by the next generation of philanthropists.*

There is, however, in response to the modern

* At the risk of weakening my argument, above, I must give a rather unique example of what, in a way, would *seem* to endorse the philanthropic position.

Richard Edwards married, first, Elizabeth Tuttle (I quote from Dr. White's *Principles of Mental Hygiene*), and later divorced her because of "adultery and other immoralities." Richard then married again, and by this second marriage had numerous descendants, none of whom became known to fame. A sister of Elizabeth committed murder, and so did a brother. *Elizabeth's grandson was Jonathan Edwards.* In 1900 (Winship), 1,394 descendants had been traced, including: 13 presidents of colleges, besides many principals of other educational institutions; 60 physicians, many of them eminent; 100 clergymen and professors; 75 officers of the army and navy; 60 prominent authors; 100 lawyers; 30 judges; and 80 holders of public office. There were no criminals.

It would seem, strictly speaking, that it is stupidity alone which is hopeless. Where there is good mental power, moral obliquity is always possible of reformation. It was with this possibility in mind that I urged the moral duty of giving *all* prisoners "a chance." This does not negative the position I have taken above as regards the older philanthropy—the cases which would fall into the Edwards' category are so few as to be almost negligible—the great majority of criminals are cases of deficient mentality, and it is absolutely sure that from them we can have none but defective descendants. To understand the Edwards' family, look back to what was said of abnormality in the opening of the Chapter on Mental Ills.

need, a new movement in philanthropy—one which concerns itself with the care of the child, and in which brotherly love is no longer allowed to obscure reason. The child and its environment are the subjects of this modern movement —the home, the health, the education, and the play of the child—and the objects are, the teaching of useful habits, the training to useful occupations, the development of community and social sense, the recognition of social duties, the formation of proper friendships, and the instilling of the more useful ideals. These are the aims of psychology, and these are the answers to the social problems which psychology can most heartily endorse. The schoolroom, the playground, the neighbourhood house, the boy and girl scout movement, and the boy and girl clubs—these are the present instruments of success.

The physical care of the child is already beginning in our larger communities, but *all* communities must be roused to its importance. The physical examinations in school should be extended to reach the whole school system, and, moreover, should be made more thorough. To the physical examination should be added psychological tests, and the mental abnormalities of the child should receive full attention. The physical defects and neuropathic tendencies, thus recognized in time, will often be found possible of correction. Nervous children, and children in the critical period, will be treated with intelligence, with an appreciation of their difficulties, and will no longer be driven, as is so often the case now, to their permanent injury. It will be remembered that it is the nervous child who is really the important member of the class; it is he who has the greatest possibilities both for good and for bad, for himself and for society. Children of bad inheritance will be especially supervised and guarded, and much at least of the harm threatened them will thus be averted.

The kindergarten should be open to all; but first to the poor. Teachers must be better prepared and, of course, better paid. The honour and dignity of the teaching profession must be more generally recognized. Educational boards must be removed from politics, and their members chosen for their knowledge of educational matters. The schools must have better sanitation, and health must be esteemed, even in the school, as superior to knowledge.

How can these happy ideals be realized? We live in a democracy, and if democracy means anything it means individual responsibility and co-operation. The church, and the school, and the state must work together. The newspapers, so many of which still warrant Ruskin's description—"the black of them coming off on your fingers and, beyond all washing, into your brains"—must cease to be textbooks of crime. Public opinion, and that means the opinion of each individual, must become active in the support of wise legislation. All must work together, and a harmonious spirit of endeavour must be created. The court, and the prison, and the police remain, but the police, in the millennium I write of, become helpful aids in securing social improvement; while the court and the prison become, respectively, the dispensary and the hospital for the treatment of social ills.

The times are urgent, the world is running amuck. War and revolution have so stirred the pool of life that all manner of horrid things have been brought to the surface. Crime and misery are rampant, and ignorance reigns supreme. New formulas in the economic field have lost their seductiveness, and basic revision of thought has become absolutely necessary.

But if the times are urgent, they are also propitious. There is now in the souls of men a spirit of public service—may it not be evanescent! Even Bolshevism, with all of its horrors, is a response to a craving for something good—its errors and misdirections are but those of crass ignorance. A great force, variously named, is seeking expression now in this world. To guide this force, and to realize its aspirations, is our duty and our only salvation. The problem is man—let man be our study.

THE END

INDEX

INDEX

285

INDEX

Conflicts, mental, 213, 225, 231
Confucius, 115
Consciousness, field of, 157
Contempt, 55
Conversion, 63
Courage, 57
Cramming, 85
Criminal, the, 266
Crowd, the, 242
Cryptopsychism, 197
Cure, nature of, 167
Curiosity, 38
Cyclic insanity, 237

Darwin, 2
Defectives, see Subnormal.
Delinquent, the, 258
Delirium, 188
Delusions, 189, 234
Dementia precox, 237
Democracy, 101, 118, 205, 255, 256, 280
Devil, the, 31
Dhyâna, 177
Disgust, 37
Dispositions, the, 6, 14, 17, 22, 37, 70
Duties of man, 259

Eddy, Mrs., 172
Education, 123
  and society, 155
  and the subconscious, 163
  difficulties of, 132, 141
  duties of parents in, 131, 134
  effect of appreciation in, 153
  effect on prejudice, 119
  effort in, 150, 155
  expectations from, 154
  individual, 156
  in former days, 126, 127
  language and, 137

of conduct, 142
of habit, 131
passivity of child in, 141
praise in, 150
present ideals of, 128
punishment in, 145
purposes of, 123, 129
results in, 154
rewards in, 149
Edwards, Jonathan, 278
Egotism, 65, 66
Élan vital, 40, 230
Elohim, 180
Emerson, 153
Emotions, classification of, 22, 57
  compound, 54
  in children and subnormal, 54
  nature of, 18, 19, 22
  simple, 22
Epictetus, 173
Epigram, the, 117

Faith, cures, see Mind cure.
  subconscious seat of, 205
Fear, 24
  effect of, on health, 167, 216
  in religion, 27
Feebleminded, the, see Subnormal.
Fielding, Henry, 270
Flammarion, 193
Fletcher, Horace, 173
Flournoy, 182, 190
Folie de doute, 222
Fore-conscious, the, 228
Forgetting, 86
Freedom of speech, 259
Freud, psychology of, 39, 216, 225

Galen, 69
Generosity, 57

286

INDEX

INDEX

INDEX

sentiments of, 66
Sufi, the, 179
Suggestion, 173
Swift, E. J., 198
Sympathy, 45
  in care of the child, 142
Syphilis and insanity, 234

Tannenbaum, Frank, 275
Telepathy, experiences in, 194
  explanations of, 193
  scientific attitude toward,
    193, 200
  testimony as to, 198
Temperament, 68
Tendencies, innate, 6, 14, 17,
    22, 37, 70
Tender emotion, 44
Thanatophobia, 223
Thought, and judgment, 103
  and language, 103
  and memory, 103, 107, 120
  and the subconscious, 118,
    201
  constructive, 108
  deliberative, 107
  in animals, 103

nature of, 103, 105
original, 108
Tramp, the, 264
Trance of cessation, 177
Trotzky, 253
Truth, 108, 110, 111
  and the subconscious, 201
  ultimate, 206

Ulysses on wisdom, 115
Unconscious, see Subconscious.
  Freud's, 228

Valedictorian, the, 127

War, 34, 52
  and spiritualism, 184
White, William A., 266, 278
Wisdom, 114
Wister, Owen, 25
Women, 44, 50
Wonder, 38
Worry, 167, 211

Yahweh, 180
Yogi, 177
Youth and age, 112